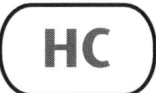

interRAI Home Care (HC) Assessment Form and User's Manual

Version 9.1

John N. Morris, PhD, MSW [Chair]
Brant E. Fries, PhD
Roberto Bernabei, MD
Knight Steel, MD
Naoki Ikegami, MD, PhD
Iain Carpenter, MD

Ruedi Gilgen, MD
Jean-Noël DuPasquier, PhD
Dinnus Frijters, PhD
Jean-Claude Henrard, MD
John P. Hirdes, PhD
Pauline Belleville-Taylor, RN, MS

interRAI Instrument and Systems Development Committee

John N. Morris, PhD, MSW [Chair]
Katherine Berg, PhD, PT
Magnus Björkgren, PhD
Dinnus Frijters, PhD
Brant E. Fries, PhD
Ruedi Gilgen, MD
Len Gray, MD, PhD
Catherine Hawes, PhD

Jean-Claude Henrard, MD
John P. Hirdes, PhD
Gunnar Ljunggren, MD, PhD
Sue Nonemaker, RN, MS
Charles D. Phillips, PhD, MPH
Knight Steel, MD
David Zimmerman, PhD

© interRAI 1994–2009
interRAI Home Care (HC)

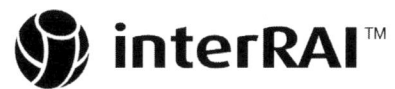

Copyright © 2009 by interRAI. Copyright © 1994, 1996, 1997, 1999, 2003, 2005, 2006 by interRAI. All rights reserved. No part of this work may be reproduced or transmitted in any form or by any means, electronic or mechanical, including photocopying and recording, or by any information storage or retrieval system without permission in writing from the publisher.

Requests for permission to reproduce material from this book should be directed to interRAI.

www.interRAI.org

Library of Congress Cataloging-in-Publication Data is available at www.loc.gov.
ISBN: 978-1-936065-00-4

Suggested Citation
Morris JN, Fries BE, Bernabei R, Steel K, Ikegami N, Carpenter I, Gilgen R, DuPasquier JN, Frijters D, Henrard JC, Hirdes JP, Belleville-Taylor P, Berg K, Björkgren M, Gray L, Hawes C, Ljunggren G, Nonemaker S, Phillips CD, Zimmerman D. interRAI Home Care (HC) Assessment Form and User's Manual, Washington, DC: interRAI, 2009.

Acknowledgments

Work on the interRAI Home Care (HC) Assessment System could not have been accomplished without the contribution and support of many people, including: Yvonne Anderson, Aleksandra Brenckle, Romanna Michajliw, Shirley Morris, and other staff at the Hebrew SeniorLife Institute for Aging Research in Boston; Nancy Curtin-Telegdi at the University of Waterloo; and staff at the CNR (Consiglio Nazionale Delle Ricerche) Target Project on Aging.

Disclaimer

Neither interRAI, the publisher, nor the authors intend that this book should be used in lieu of comprehensive appropriate care. Every reasonable effort has been made to ensure that the information provided is accurate and up to date. However, the person's physician or other authorized practitioner should validate information about drugs and therapies for appropriateness before prescribing.

For information or comments on the interRAI Home Care (HC) Assessment System, visit www.interRAI.org.

Development of the interRAI Home Care (HC) Assessment System and Related Materials

A multinational group of clinicians and researchers, consisting of interRAI Fellows, began work on Version 1 of the RAI HC in 1993. Several updates of Version 1 were released between 1994 and 1997—including Version 1.7, Version 1.10a, and Version 1.11. These instruments were used extensively in North America, Europe, and Asia.

A major revision and update of the entire system was released as "Version 2.0" in 1999. A few items were deleted, several items modified, and a few items added. The basic time frame for an assessment was reduced from 7 days to 3 days (where possible). Triggers were streamlined and text updated in most of the thirty Clinical Assessment Protocols (CAPs).

In 2001, interRAI began a restructuring initiative to ensure that all instruments contained common items and definitions. This major revision of the home care instrument is known as the interRAI HC Assessment.

Although not included in this user's manual, a variety of support materials are available. These include: (1) standardized scoring schema for creating summary indicators for measures such as ADLs, Cognition, Communication, Pain, and Mood; (2) a screening system to identify appropriate care pathways for persons (the MI-Choice© system); (3) a case-mix system that places persons into distinct service-use/intensity categories (RUG-III/HC); (4) translations of the interRAI HC Assessment System into several languages other than English; and (5) a variety of software systems to facilitate data entry and triggering of the CAPs.

We also note that the interRAI HC Assessment System is one of a series of integrated assessment tools that interRAI maintains to assess and monitor the status of a person with needs for care. Other assessment and problem identification tools include the interRAI LTCF Assessment System for nursing home and long-term care institutional settings, the interRAI PAC Assessment System for post-acute care, the interRAI MH Assessment System for institutional mental health care, the interRAI CMH Assessment System for community mental health care, the interRAI PC Assessment System for palliative care, the interRAI AC Assessment System for acute hospital care, and the interRAI ID Assessment System for the care of persons with intellectual disabilities.

Contents

Part I   **About the interRAI Home Care (HC) Assessment System**   1

       Introduction   1

       Approaching the interRAI Home Care (HC) Assessment System   2

Part II   **Item-by-Item Guide to the interRAI Home Care (HC) Assessment Form**   7

       Section A. Identification Information   9

       Section B. Intake and Initial History   17

       Section C. Cognition   19

       Section D. Communication and Vision   25

       Section E. Mood and Behavior   29

       Section F. Psychosocial Well-Being   35

       Section G. Functional Status   39

       Section H. Continence   51

       Section I. Disease Diagnoses   55

       Section J. Health Conditions   59

       Section K. Oral and Nutritional Status   69

       Section L. Skin Condition   73

       Section M. Medications   77

       Section N. Treatments and Procedures   89

       Section O. Responsibility   95

       Section P. Social Supports   97

       Section Q. Environmental Assessment   101

       Section R. Discharge Potential and Overall Status   103

       Section S. Discharge   105

       Section T. Assessment Information   107

Appendices

       List of Abbreviations   109

       interRAI Home Care (HC) Assessment Form

Part I

About the interRAI Home Care (HC) Assessment System

Introduction

Throughout the world, people are living longer and the birthrate is falling. The population of persons over the age of 65 is rapidly growing, both in raw numbers and as a proportion of the whole. For example, for the first time in Italy's history, there are more persons over age 65 than under age 20. In most developed countries the increase is particularly striking for those aged 80 and older. Improving the ability of the health care delivery system to respond to the needs of those requiring community-based care in a fiscally responsible manner is one of the greatest challenges of our times.

The interRAI Home Care (HC) Assessment System

The interRAI HC Assessment System has been designed to be a user-friendly, reliable, person-centered system that informs and guides comprehensive planning of care and services in community-based settings around the world. It focuses on the person's functioning and quality of life by assessing needs, strengths, and preferences. It also facilitates referrals when appropriate. When used on multiple occasions, it provides the basis for an outcome-based assessment of the person's response to care or services. The interRAI HC Assessment System can be used to assess persons with chronic needs for care, as well as those with post-acute care needs (for example, after hospitalization or in a hospital-at-home situation). The interRAI HC Assessment System has been designed to be compatible with the suite of interRAI assessment and problem-identification tools. Such compatibility advances continuity of care through a "seamless" assessment system across multiple health care settings, and promotes a person-centered evaluation rather than fragmented site-specific assessments.

The interRAI HC Assessment System consists of the interRAI HC Assessment Form; this manual, which shows you how to use the Assessment Form; and the Clinical Assessment Protocols (CAPs).

The interRAI HC Assessment Form is a Minimum Data Set (MDS) screening tool that enables a home care provider to assess multiple key domains of function, health, social support, and service use. Particular interRAI HC items also identify persons who could benefit from further evaluation of specific problems or risks for functional decline. These items, known as "triggers," link the interRAI HC to a series of problem-oriented CAPs.

The Clinical Assessment Protocols (CAPs) contain general guidelines for further assessment and individualized care and services. There are thirty CAPs in multiple domains (including clinical, mental health, psychosocial, and physical function). On average, a person receiving home care services triggers about ten of the thirty CAPs. Your goal is to use this information to arrive at an appropriate plan of care, and where possible and required, provide the service or make a referral. At the same time, we recognize that home care professionals may be operating within a program where reimbursement systems or eligibility requirements limit their care options. You may not be able to offer home care services to address all problem areas. Nevertheless, a comprehensive assessment that includes the strengths and needs of the person can be useful as you schedule services and assess program outcomes.

Government agencies from around the world have adopted the interRAI HC Assessment System, either in its entirety (with or without country-specific supplemental items) or with slight local modifications. A number of private organizations and agencies are also using the interRAI HC Assessment System.

Approaching the interRAI Home Care (HC) Assessment System

This manual provides information to facilitate an accurate and uniform assessment of persons served by community-based programs—home care, board and care, assisted living, etc.

Use of the interRAI HC Assessment Form

The interRAI HC Assessment Form is a standardized, minimal assessment and screening tool designed for clinical use. It is not a questionnaire for analyzing the characteristics of a population, nor does it include all the information that might be necessary to construct a comprehensive plan of care. Supplemental information, relevant to the person, should be assessed and incorporated as necessary. The items in the interRAI HC measure a person's objective performance and capacity in a variety of areas, with the majority of items serving as triggers for specific CAPs.

Key points regarding completion of the interRAI HC assessment follow:

- The interRAI HC Assessment System is designed for use by clinical professionals (nurses, social workers, physicians, therapists, etc.). With appropriate training, however, individuals without a clinical background can generally perform an accurate assessment. While there are no requirements regarding who performs the assessment, the provider agency is responsible for implementing a quality assurance system to ensure the accuracy of assessments.

- The interRAI HC Assessment Form consists of items and definitions. It should be used as a guide to structure a clinical and social assessment in planning for community-based care and services.

- The assessment process requires communication with the person and primary caregiver/family member (if available), observation of the person in the home environment, and review of secondary documents when available. Where possible, the person is the primary source of information.

- Items on the interRAI HC Assessment Form flow in a logical sequence and can be completed in the order in which they appear. However, the assessor is not bound by this sequence. Items may be reviewed in any order that works for the assessor and the person. For additional ideas on how to sequence the assessment, see "Initiating the interRAI HC Assessment Process" on page 4.

- Sometimes the assessor must reconcile multiple sources of information yielding seemingly inconsistent results (for example, the person being assessed may report something that is very different from the response of the person's daughter). In this case, the assessor must use his or her clinical judgment to determine the most appropriate response for the particular item(s).

- Assessors should talk in private with each informant, if possible.

- Whenever possible, the assessment should be performed in the person's home. Parts of the assessment can be completed in settings other than the person's home (such as a hospital, day care center, or outpatient clinic) with no loss in information quality. However, certain critical items (such as environmental factors) can best be assessed in the home.

- The initial interRAI HC assessment should be completed when the person is first referred for service by an agency. Subsequent assessments should be completed according to the schedule prescribed by your agency.

Introducing the Person to the interRAI HC Assessment Process

In introducing the interRAI HC assessment to a person, you will normally be dealing with someone who has applied for or is eligible for a home-based program of care. You should emphasize that the assessment is an integral part of the overall service program. If service options are limited, be realistic in channeling the conversation.

Address the person directly whenever possible. When talking with others, it is not necessary to use the word "person," which is used on the interRAI HC Assessment Form to provide a consistent reference throughout. You can substitute words such as "older adult," "patient," or "client." You can also use phrases such as "Mrs. X" or "your mother."

Basic Principles of the interRAI HC Assessment Process

- You are a guest in the person's home.
- Your purpose is to complete a comprehensive assessment of the person, with the goal of:
  - Maximizing the individual's functional capacity and quality of life;
  - Addressing health problems; and
  - Ensuring that the individual remains in his or her home as long as possible.
- To do this requires:
  - Identifying the purpose of your visit;
  - Identifying functional, medical, and social issues that are presently limiting or likely will become limiting;
  - Identifying the person's strengths and assets; and
  - Integrating what you see and hear in order to accurately code each of the interRAI HC Assessment items.
- Information collected using the interRAI HC can serve to:
  - Provide a basis for further evaluation of unrecognized or unmet needs; and
  - Develop a care plan that ensures that each limiting or potentially limiting factor is both viewed in the context of the life circumstances unique to that individual and managed so as to maximize that person's quality of life and function.

- Do not expect that all functional, medical, and social matters you identify will be fully and comprehensively addressed during your initial visit. Rather, it is more important that all major functional, medical, and social circumstances that limit the individual's quality of life be identified in order to develop a plan for further evaluation or management.
- Any acute medical matter should be brought to the attention of the person immediately, and the person should be vigorously counseled to seek appropriate medical care, whether or not that can be provided in the home setting.
- If there is evidence of abuse or neglect, referral to an appropriate agency/authority and immediate intervention may be warranted, in accordance with the laws of your local jurisdiction.

Initiating the interRAI HC Assessment Process

Icebreaker questions. You can begin the assessment process with a series of optional "icebreaker" questions that will serve to begin a dialogue with the person and family, and may begin to elicit much of the information required to complete the assessment. These questions are not listed on the assessment form; they can vary by country/local custom or depending on whether this is an initial or follow-up assessment. Some examples:

- How are you (is the person) doing? How do you (does he/she) get around in the house?
- How do you (does the person) perceive your (his/her) present health as compared to a year ago (or when last seen)?
- Do you (does the person) feel well enough to do what you want (he/she wants) to do?
- Can you (can the person) do the things that you want (he/she wants) to do? What type of assistance or services do you (does the person) need?

Structuring the order of the assessment. When conducting an assessment in a person's home, the assessor needs to consider the order in which the items in the assessment will be addressed. It is generally helpful to assess the person's cognitive status and ability to communicate early on, so that you can gauge the reliability of the information you are gathering from the person. There is also a need to be sensitive to the person's reaction to the assessment process and particular issues. There is no one right order in which the sections of the interRAI HC should be addressed. Take your follow-up cues from the person's responses to the "icebreaker" questions for prioritizing areas for assessment. Remember, this is not a questionnaire—the person's needs should set the pace and priorities for the assessment process, although you must gather all the information necessary to complete the interRAI HC Assessment. More than one interview with the person or follow-up contacts with family members, other caregivers, or the person's physician may be necessary.

How to Use this Manual

Use this manual alongside the interRAI HC Assessment Form, keeping the form in front of you at all times. The Assessment Form itself contains a wealth of information. Learn to rely on the form until you internalize the item definitions and procedural instructions necessary for accurate assessment. The amplifying information in this manual should be reviewed in total prior to completing your first interRAI HC assessment. Then keep the manual handy so that you can continue to refer to it as questions arise during the completion of subsequent assessments. The initial time investment in this multistep review process will have a major payback.

The guidelines that follow summarize our recommended approach to becoming familiar with the interRAI HC assessment process.

Becoming Familiar with the interRAI HC Assessment Process

First, review the interRAI HC Assessment Form itself.

- Notice how sections are organized and where information is to be recorded.
- If you previously worked with MDS-HC Version 2.0 or with earlier versions of the interRAI HC Assessment Form, begin by reviewing the form for new items and changes in codes.
- Work through one section at a time. Examine item definitions and response options. Review procedural instructions, time frames, and general coding conventions.
- Are the item definitions and instructions clear? Do they differ from your agency's current practice? What areas require further clarification?

Next, complete a sample interRAI HC Assessment for a person in your program.

- Draw only on your existing knowledge of this individual. Enter the appropriate codes on the interRAI HC Assessment Form.
- Note where your assessment could benefit from additional information. How might you secure specific information? By asking the person? By talking with the family?

Next, complete an initial pass through Part II, "Item-by-Item Guide to the interRAI Home Care (HC) Assessment Form".

- Part II includes:
  - The intent of items on the interRAI HC Assessment Form;
  - Supplemental definitions and instructions for completing interRAI HC items;
  - Reminders of which items refer to a time frame for observing the person other than the standard **3-day** observation period generally used throughout the assessment instrument; and
  - Sources of information to be consulted for specific items.
- As you read the item definitions, review questions that arose as you used the interRAI HC Assessment for the first time to assess a person. Note sections of this manual that help to clarify any coding and procedural questions you may have had.
- Read the instructions that apply to each section of the interRAI HC Assessment Form. Make sure you understand the information before going on to another section. Review the test case you completed. Would you still code it the same? It will take time to go through all this material. Do not rush. Work through the interRAI HC Assessment one section at a time to make sure you thoroughly understand the definitions and instructions.

- Are you surprised by any of the interRAI HC item definitions, instructions, or case examples? For example, do you understand how to code "activities of daily living" (ADLs)? Or "mood"?
- Do any definitions or instructions differ from what you thought you learned when you first reviewed the interRAI HC Assessment Form? Would you now complete your initial case differently?
- Do any item definitions or instructions differ from current practice patterns or terminology used in your agency?
- Make notations next to anything you have questions about. Be prepared to discuss these issues during any formal training program you attend.

Future use of information in this manual:

- Keep this manual at hand during the assessment process.
- Where necessary, review the intent of each item in question.
- This manual will serve as a reference as long as you are using the interRAI HC Assessment Form. Use it on an ongoing basis to increase the accuracy of your assessments.

Part II

Item-by-Item Guide to the interRAI Home Care (HC) Assessment Form

To facilitate completion of the interRAI HC Assessment and to ensure consistent interpretation of items, this chapter presents the following types of information for many (**but not all**) items:

Intent — Reason(s) for including the item (or set of items) in the interRAI HC Assessment, including discussions of how the information will be used by clinical staff to identify problems and develop a plan of care.

Definition — Explanation of key terms.

Process — Sources of information and methods for determining the correct response for an item. Sources include:

- Interview and observation of the person;
- Discussion with the person's family, other caregivers, and the person's physician; and
- Review of any clinical records or other administrative documentation.

Coding — Proper method of recording the response for each item, with explanations of the individual response options.

This item-by-item guide follows the sequence of items on the interRAI HC Assessment Form.

Section A

Identification Information

Intent — This section contains personal identifiers necessary to identify the person and link sequential assessments in an electronic database.

A1. Name

Definition — Person's legal name.

Coding — Use printed letters. Enter in the following order:

- **A1a.** First name
- **A1b.** Middle initial
- **A1c.** Last name (surname/family name)
- **A1d.** Jr./Sr.

If the person has no middle initial, leave Item A1b blank. Likewise, leave Item A1d blank if appropriate.

A2. Gender

Coding
1. Male
2. Female

A3. Birthdate

Coding — For the month and day of date of birth, enter two digits each. Use a leading zero ("0") as a filler if a single digit. Use four digits for the year. Example: November 1, 1942.

1	9	4	2		1	1		0	1
Year					Month			Day	

A4. Marital Status

Coding — Choose the answer that describes the current marital status of the person. If the person is in a common-law relationship, score the item **"2"** for "Married". If the person is in a same-sex relationship that is legally recognized as a marriage, score the item **"2"** for "Married". If the person is in a long-term same-sex relationship that is not legally recognized as a marriage, score the item **"3"** for "Partner/significant other".

1. Never married
2. Married
3. Partner/significant other
4. Widowed
5. Separated
6. Divorced

A5. National Numeric Identifier [Country Specific]

NOTE: If not in the USA, please consult your addendum.

Intent To record personal identification numbers.

Process Ask the person and caregiver for permission to review any existing personal records that contain relevant information. If you cannot obtain this information, consult with your agency's business office on how to proceed.

Coding Begin writing one number per box, starting with the box farthest to the left. Recheck the number to be sure you have written the digits correctly.

A5a. **Social Security number** — Enter the person's Social Security number. If the person does not have a Social Security number (for example, if the person is a recent immigrant or a child), leave blank.

A5b. **Medicare number (or comparable railroad insurance number)** — Enter the person's Medicare number. Approximately 98% of people aged 65 or older in the United States have a Medicare number. This number occasionally changes based on marital status. If a question arises, check with your agency's business office or social worker.

In rare instances, the person will have neither a Medicare number nor a Social Security number. When this occurs, another type of basic identification number (for example, railroad retirement insurance number) may be substituted. In such cases, place a "C" in the left-most Medicare number scoring box; then, starting with the second box, continue entering the number itself, one digit per box. Enter "N" if the person has neither a Medicare or railroad retirement insurance number.

A5c. **Medicaid number** — Enter the person's Medicaid number. Enter "+" if the number is pending, and "N" if the person is not on Medicaid.

A6. Facility/Agency Provider Number

Intent To be able to track the provider of services.

Process Enter the number assigned to your agency. In the U.S., Medicare or the State may assign this number.

Coding Begin writing one digit per box, starting with the left-most box. Recheck the number to be sure you have written the digits correctly.

A7. Current Payment Sources [Country Specific]

NOTE: If not in the USA, please consult your addendum.

Intent   To document the sources of payment for home care services.

Definitions
- **A7a. Medicaid** — Pays for nursing care and other necessary therapies or services.
- **A7b. Medicare** — Pays for nursing care and other necessary therapies or services.
- **A7c. Self or family pays for full per diem cost** — The person or family pays the full cost of care and services.
- **A7d. Medicare with Medicaid co-payment** — The State is responsible for the Medicare co-payment by way of Medicaid.
- **A7e. Private insurance** — The person's private insurance company (for example, a company providing long-term care insurance) covers all or part of the cost of care and services.
- **A7f. Other per diem** — Another entity covers all or part of the cost of care and services.

Process   Consult with business or billing office to review payment sources used within the last 30 days. Do not rely exclusively on information recorded in the person's service record (usually the face sheet at the front of the administrative or clinical record), as sources of payment may change while receiving services, based on the person's condition. Capture all methods of payment.

Coding   Enter "1" for payors of services in the last 30 days; enter "0" for all others. **Note: Billing office to provide this information.**

0. No
1. Yes

A8. Reason for Assessment

Intent   To document the reason for completing the assessment.

Coding   Enter the number corresponding to the reason for assessment.

1. **First assessment** — An assessment that is done at the time of entry into the home care system, or when initially determining eligibility for home care/home health services.

2. **Routine reassessment** — A regularly scheduled follow-up assessment to ensure that the care plan is appropriate and current.

3. **Return assessment** — An assessment conducted when the person returns from the hospital or re-enters the home care system after a planned absence.

4. **Significant change in status reassessment** — A comprehensive reassessment conducted at any time during the uninterrupted course of care because the person's status or condition has significantly changed. If the change in status is accompanied by a hospital stay, code "3" for "Return assessment" instead.

5. **Discharge assessment, covers last 3 days of service** — Use this code whenever a permanent program discharge is anticipated and a full interRAI HC Assessment

is completed. This is a means of "closing" the clinical record at the point of discharge. Your agency or home care program will determine the type of discharge assessment to be completed (discharge assessment or discharge tracking only).

6. Discharge tracking only — Use this code when the person is discharged from the home care service without a full interRAI HC assessment being completed. Discharge tracking items are completed to indicate within a data system that the person is no longer receiving service from the home care program. Examples include death, admission to an extended-stay facility, or a hospitalization when return to the home care service is not anticipated.

7. Other — For example, research. Any assessment conducted outside of the established assessment schedule for reasons such as quality assurance, clinical research, confirmation of the appropriateness of the current plan (not the routine "follow-up" reassessment), development of acuity scale, community needs assessment, etc.

A9. Assessment Reference Date

Intent

To establish a common period of observation as a reference point for each completed assessment.

Definition

The designated end point of the common observation period for items on the interRAI HC. Except where otherwise noted, all information gathered about the person pertains to the 3-day period prior to and including the Assessment Reference Date for items pertaining to the person's status or performance. Home care assessments are usually completed using information gathered during a single visit. However, when an assessment carries over to a second visit, information for the remaining interRAI HC items must be for the time period established by the original Assessment Reference Date. In other words, although the assessor may visit the person on different dates, the coding for all items completed on subsequent visits refers to the person's status during the time period for the Assessment Reference Date established on the initial visit.

Coding

For the month and day of the assessment, enter two digits each. Use a leading zero ("0") as a filler if a single digit. Use four digits for the year. Example: May 8, 2005. The period of observation for 3-day items includes May 6–8.

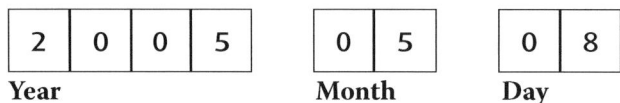

Year | Month | Day
2 0 0 5 | 0 5 | 0 8

A10. Person's Expressed Goals of Care

Intent

The person being assessed is an important member of the health care team. It is essential to ask him or her to identify what his or her goals of care might be. By doing so, the assessor encourages the person to be an active member of the team. This can also be a starting point to develop a person-centered plan of care or services.

Process

Use this box to document outcomes that the person hopes to achieve as a result of receiving services. These outcomes may relate to almost anything, including improved functional performance, a return to health, increased independence, an ability to maintain community residence, improved social relations, etc.

Talk to the person and phrase your questions about goals of care in the most general way possible. For example, ask: "How can we help you?" "Why are you getting (or applying for) services?" "What benefits do you expect to get?" "What changes in yourself do you hope will occur?" Encourage the person to express personal goals in his or her own words.

Some persons will be unable to articulate a goal, an expected outcome, or even a reason for seeking services. They may say they do not know or that they are getting service at the request of a relative. All of these are reasonable responses. Do not make inferences based on what you or other clinicians believe **should** be goals of care. If the person asks you for clarification on what he or she might expect from services, follow your usual agency policy.

Coding Use the large ("open text") box to record the person's verbatim response. Code the person's primary goal of care in the single line of boxes at the bottom, entering one letter in each box. Abbreviate if necessary. Enter "NONE" if the person is unable to articulate a goal of care.

| B | E | S | U | R | E | I | T | A | K | E | M | E | D | S |

A11. Postal/Zip Code of Usual Living Arrangement [Country Specific]

NOTE: If not in the USA, please consult your addendum.

Definition The postal or zip code for the community address where the person usually resides. For those persons being evaluated while in an acute care hospital, rehabilitation hospital or unit, post acute unit, or nursing home, this would be the community address of the person's usual living arrangement prior to his or her stay in the current institutional setting.

Process Talk to the person or family member. Review the person's admission or transmittal records as necessary.

Coding Enter one digit per box, beginning with the left-most box. If the four-digit code extension is unavailable, leave the extra four digits blank. For example, Roslindale, MA 02131 should be entered as follows:

| 0 | 2 | 1 | 3 | 1 | – | | | | |

A12. Residential/Living Status at Time of Assessment

Intent To document the person's living arrangement at the time of the current assessment. The person's living arrangement may be long-standing or temporary.

Process Ask the person or family if you are unsure of where the person is currently living, or consult the person's administrative records.

Coding Choose only one answer and enter the appropriate code in the box provided. If the code is a single digit, leave the first box empty.

1. **Private home/apartment/rented room** — Any house, condominium, apartment, or room in the community, whether owned or rented by the person or

another party. Also included in this category are retirement communities and independent housing for older adults or the disabled.

2. **Board and care** — A noninstitutional community residential setting that integrates a shared living environment with varying degrees of supportive services of the following types: supervision, home health, homemaker, personal care, meal service, transportation, etc.

3. **Assisted living or semi-independent living** — A second type of noninstitutional community residential setting that integrates a shared living environment with varying degrees of supportive services of the following types: supervision, home health, homemaker, personal care, meal service, transportation, etc.

4. **Mental health residence** — e.g., psychiatric group home. A residential setting for adults with mental health problems who need supervision and limited services (meals, housekeeping).

5. **Group home for persons with physical disability** — A setting that provides services to persons with physical disabilities. Typically, persons live in group settings with 24-hour staff presence. Individuals are encouraged to be as independent and active as possible.

6. **Setting for persons with intellectual disability** — A setting that provides services to persons with intellectual disabilities. Typically, persons live in group settings with 24-hour staff presence, but are encouraged to be as independent and active as possible.

7. **Psychiatric hospital or unit** — A psychiatric hospital that focuses on the diagnosis and treatment of psychiatric disorders and which is separate from other inpatient facilities, such as an acute care, rehabilitation, or chronic care hospital. A psychiatric unit is a single unit, located in a general hospital, which is dedicated to the diagnosis and treatment of psychiatric disorders.

8. **Homeless (with or without shelter)** — A homeless person does not have a fixed residence (a house, apartment, room, or other place to stay on a regular basis). The person may live on the streets, or outside in wooded or open areas. The person may sleep in cars, in abandoned buildings, under bridges, etc. Persons who are homeless may or may not take advantage of existing homeless shelters.

9. **Long-term care facility (nursing home)** — A licensed health care facility that provides 24-hour skilled or intermediate-level nursing care.

10. **Rehabilitation hospital/unit** — A licensed rehabilitation hospital that focuses on the physical and occupational rehabilitation of individuals who have experienced disease or injury with subsequent decline in physical function. A rehabilitation unit is located within an acute care hospital and focuses on the acute rehabilitation of individuals who have experienced disease or injury with a subsequent decline in physical function.

11. **Hospice facility/palliative care unit** — A hospice facility (or unit within a facility providing more general care) provides care to persons who have a terminal illness with a prognosis of less than 6 months to live as certified by a physician. The goal of hospice care is to provide comfort and quality of life while assisting the person and family. Palliative care is the care of persons whose diseases are not responsive to curative treatments. It targets pain and symptom relief, without precluding use of life-prolonging treatments. Palliative care is often provided from the time a person is diagnosed with a life-threatening illness.

12. **Acute care hospital** — A facility licensed as an acute care hospital that focuses primarily on the diagnosis and treatment of acute medical disorders.

13. **Correctional facility** — Any jail, penitentiary, or halfway house operated by a local, state, or federal government to care for and house persons who have been sentenced to incarceration by a criminal court.

14. **Other** — Any other type of setting not listed above.

A13. Living Arrangement

Intent To record whom the person lives with and the duration of this arrangement. These items will help the home care staff determine the need for more, fewer, or different services.

Process Ask the person or family member.

A13a. Lives

Coding Record the code that reflects whom the person is living with presently. Note that this excludes any temporary arrangements in living made while home care services are being set up. Choose only one answer and enter the appropriate code in the box provided.

1. **Alone** — Includes person who lives only with a pet, lives on the streets, or is homeless (whether or not the person uses shelters).

2. **With spouse/partner only** — Includes spouse/partner, girlfriend or boyfriend, common-law marriage, or long-term same-sex relationship.

3. **With spouse/partner and other(s)** — Lives with spouse or partner and any other individual(s), whether family or unrelated.

4. **With child (not spouse/partner)** — Lives with child(ren) only, or with child(ren) and other individual(s), but **not** with spouse or partner.

5. **With parent(s) or guardian(s)** — Lives with parent(s) or guardian(s) only, or with parent(s) or guardian(s) and other individual(s), but **not** with spouse or partner or child(ren).

6. **With sibling(s)** — Lives with sibling(s) only, or with sibling(s) and other individual(s), but **not** with spouse or partner, child(ren), or parent(s) or guardian(s).

7. **With other relative(s)** — Lives with a relative (such as aunt or uncle) other than spouse or partner, child(ren), parent(s), or sibling(s).

8. **With nonrelative(s)** — Lives in a group setting (for example, a boarding home, long-term care facility, group home, or jail) or in shared accommodation with nonrelative(s) (for example, roommate). Excludes single overnight stays, such as in a homeless shelter.

A13b.	**As compared to 90 DAYS AGO (or since last assessment), person now lives with someone new**
Definition	This item indicates whether a person's living situation has changed in the last 90 days. For example, the person has moved in with another person; someone else has moved in with the person; or the person's spouse has died in the last 90 days.

A13c.	**Person or relative feels the person would be better off living elsewhere**
Process	Ask the person and family member/caregiver separately whether either believes there should be a change in living arrangements. Be sensitive to how the question is raised. Variants on the question "Do you believe the person would be better off living elsewhere?" might include asking whether the person would be happier/less isolated living elsewhere, would have his or her needs met better, would be safer, or would have access to more nutritious meals.
Coding	Code for the most appropriate response. 0. No 1. Yes, other community residence 2. Yes, institution

A14. Time Since Last Hospital Stay

Intent	To document the time of the most recent instance of hospitalization during the last 90 days. This information can be useful in assessing the stability of the person's condition(s) and whether post acute care is needed.
Process	Ask the person how long it has been since he or she was last discharged from an inpatient hospital setting. Calculate the period counting back from the Assessment Reference Date.
Coding	Code for the most recent instance in the **last 90 days**. 0. No hospitalization within 90 days 1. 31 to 90 days ago 2. 15 to 30 days ago 3. 8 to 14 days ago 4. In the last 7 days 5. Now in hospital

Section B

Intake and Initial History

NOTE: This section is completed only when the person is admitted to the home care service or when the first interRAI HC Assessment is completed. It provides basic information about the person that is not expected to change during the person's involvement with the service.

B1. Date Case Opened (This Agency)

Intent To document the date the person's case was initiated by the agency or service.

Process Enter the date when the person was first referred to the agency or service. If the care agency did not receive a referral, enter the date when the person first became known to the agency as needing an interRAI HC Assessment. If the person were transferred from another agency, the date would be the date of transfer. The record is likely to be the most reliable source of this information.

Coding Fill in the boxes with the appropriate number. Do not leave any boxes blank. If the month or day contains only a single digit, fill the first box with a "0". For example, if the care agency received a referral from the primary care provider on March 14, 2005, the date should be entered as:

2	0	0	5		0	3		1	4
Year					Month			Day	

B2. Ethnicity and Race [Country Specific]

NOTE: If not in the USA, please consult your addendum.

Intent To document the person's race and ethnicity per established standards.

Process Ask the person or family member which of the categories below best describes their race and ethnic background. The person may identify more than one category.

Coding For each option that applies, enter **"1"** for "Yes". For options that do not apply, enter **"0"** for "No".

Ethnicity

B2a. Hispanic or Latino

Race

B2b. American Indian or Alaska Native

B2c. Asian

B2d. Black or African American

B2e. Native Hawaiian or other Pacific Islander
B2f. White

B3. Primary Language [Country Specific]

NOTE: If not in the USA, please consult your addendum.

Intent
To record the person's preferred language for day-to-day communication. Caregivers and other staff must be able to communicate with the person in a language he or she understands. Information about the person's language may indicate the need to consider interpretation services.

Definition
Preferred language for day-to-day communication.

Process
Observe and interview the person and family to determine the language the person primarily speaks or understands. Review any clinical records.

Coding
Code for the most appropriate category.

1. English
2. Spanish
3. French
4. Other

B4. Residential History over Last 5 Years

Process
Ask the person and caregivers. Review any available documentation.

Definitions

B4a. **Long-term care facility** — For example, nursing home. A licensed health care facility that provides 24-hour skilled or intermediate-level nursing care.

B4b. **Board and care home, assisted living** — A noninstitutional community residential setting that integrates a shared living environment with varying degrees of supportive services of the following types: supervision, meal service, transportation, etc.

B4c. **Mental health residence** — For example, psychiatric group home. A residential setting for adults with mental health problems who need supervision and limited services (meals, housekeeping).

B4d. **Psychiatric hospital or unit** — A hospital that focuses on the diagnosis and treatment of psychiatric disorders and which is separate from other inpatient facilities, such as an acute, rehabilitation or chronic hospital. A psychiatric unit is a single unit, located in a general hospital, which is dedicated to the diagnosis and treatment of psychiatric disorders.

B4e. **Setting for persons with intellectual disability** — A setting that provides services to persons with intellectual disabilities. Typically, such persons live in group settings with 24-hour staff presence. Persons are encouraged to be as independent and active as possible.

Coding
Code for all settings the person lived in during the **5 years** prior to the date the case was opened (Item B1).

0. No
1. Yes

Section C
Cognition

It is important to determine the person's actual performance in remembering, making decisions, and organizing daily self-care activities. These items are crucial factors in many care planning decisions, in part because of their impact upon the person's ability to follow instructions and treatment regimens, and to make independent decisions in the community.

C1. Cognitive Skills for Daily Decision Making

Intent

To record the person's actual performance in making everyday decisions about the tasks or activities of daily living. These items are especially important for further assessment and care planning in that they can alert the assessor to a mismatch between a person's abilities and his or her current level of performance, as the family may inadvertently be fostering the person's dependence.

Definition

Here are some examples of decision-making tasks:

- Choosing items of clothing
- Knowing when to eat meals
- Knowing and using space in the home appropriately
- Using environmental cues (such as clocks or calendars) to organize and plan the day
- In the absence of environmental cues, seeking information appropriately (i.e., not repetitively) from family in order to plan the day
- Using awareness of one's own strengths and limitations in regulating the day's events (for example, asking for help when necessary)
- Making prudent decisions concerning how and when to go out of the house; where applicable, acknowledging the need to use a walker or other assistive device and using it faithfully

Process

Interview and observe the person, then consult with a family member or other caregiver. Review the events of each day. **The inquiry should focus on whether the person is actively making decisions about how to manage tasks of daily living, and not whether the caregiver believes that the person might be capable of doing so. Remember that the intent of this item is to record what the person is doing (actual performance).** When a family member takes decision-making responsibility away from the person regarding tasks of everyday living, or when the person chooses not to participate in decision making (whatever his or her level of capability may be), the person should be considered as having impaired performance in decision making.

Coding

Enter the single number that corresponds to the most correct response. If the person receives a score of **"5"**, do not complete the rest of Section C or any of Sections D, E, or F; instead, skip directly to Section G.

0. **Independent** — The person's decisions in organizing daily routines and making decisions were consistent, reasonable, and safe (reflecting life-style, culture, values).

1. **Modified independence** — The person organized daily routines and made safe decisions in familiar situations, but experienced some difficulty in decision making when faced with **new** tasks or situations **only**.

2. **Minimally impaired** — In specific recurring situations, decisions were poor or unsafe, with cues/supervision necessary at those times.

3. **Moderately impaired** — The person's decisions were consistently poor or unsafe; the person required reminders, cues, or supervision at all times to plan, organize, and conduct daily routines.

4. **Severely impaired** — The person never (or rarely) made decisions.

5. **No discernable consciousness, coma** — The person is nonresponsive. (Skip to Section G.)

C2. Memory/Recall Ability

NOTE: If the person received a score of "5" ("No discernable consciousness, coma") on Item C1, do not complete Items C2–C5 or any of the items in Section D, Section E, or Section F. Instead, proceed directly to Section G.

Intent

To determine a person's ability to remember recent and past events (short-term and situational memory) and to perform sequential activities (procedural memory).

Definitions

C2a. **Short-term memory OK** — Seems, appears to recall after 5 minutes.

C2b. **Procedural memory OK** — Can perform all or almost all steps in a multi-task sequence without cues.

C2c. **Situational memory OK** — Both recognizes the names/faces of caregivers frequently encountered and knows the location of places regularly visited (bedroom, kitchen, etc.).

Process

C2a. **Short-term memory OK** — Conduct a structured test of short-term memory (for the preferred approach, see the following "Example"). If this is not possible, ask the person to describe a recent event that you should both have knowledge of (for example, the election of a new political leader, a major holiday) or that you can validate with a family member (for example, what the person had for breakfast). **If there is no positive indication of memory ability, score this item "1" for "Memory problem".**

C2b. **Procedural memory OK** — This item refers to the cognitive ability needed to perform sequential activities. Dressing is an example of such an activity, as multiple steps are required to complete the entire task. The person must be able to perform or remember to perform all or most of the steps in order to be scored **"0"** for "Memory OK". If the person demonstrates difficulty in two or more steps, code as **"1"** for "Memory problem". Remember that persons in need of care in the home often have physical limitations that impede their independent performance of activities. Do not confuse such physical limitations with the cognitive ability (or inability) to perform sequential activities.

> **Example of a Structured Approach for Assessing Short-Term Memory**
>
> Ask the person to remember three unrelated items (such as book, watch, and table) for a few minutes. After you have stated all three items, ask the person to repeat them to you (to verify that you were heard and understood by the person). Then proceed to talk about something else, perhaps by going on to another part of the assessment. Do not be silent; do not leave the room. In 5 minutes, ask the person to repeat the name of each item. For persons with verbal communication deficits, nonverbal responses are acceptable (for example, when asked to point to items that are to be recalled, he or she can do so). **If the person is unable to recall all three items, Item C2a should be scored "1" for "Memory problem".**

C2c. **Situational memory OK** — This two-part measure of orientation assesses the person's cognitive ability to recognize both people and places. To be coded as OK, the person must **both** recognize the names/faces of frequently encountered family members or caregivers **and** know the location of places regularly visited (bedroom, dining room, places visited outside the home). It is not necessary for the person to know the street number of the house or apartment, but he or she should be able to find the way to his or her room, recognize the purposes of particular rooms, etc.

Coding   For C2a, C2b, and C2c, code for recall of what was learned or known.

NOTE: When you are coding C2c, the person must demonstrate positive abilities in BOTH types of situations (i.e., caregiver names/faces AND locations) to be coded as "0". If the person demonstrates difficulty in one or both areas, code **"1"** for "Memory problem".

0. **Yes, memory OK**

1. **Memory problem**

> **Examples of How to Code Memory/Recall Ability**
>
> Mrs. L is a 90-year-old former librarian who became a home care client 2 days ago, after being discharged from a rehabilitation hospital for continued occupational and physical therapy following surgical repair of a hip fracture. During the assessment Mrs. L was articulate about her recent health history (including the names of the acute and rehabilitation hospitals, orthopedic surgeon, and primary nurses). She enumerated her current medication list and when the medications were to be taken, and reported that she did this activity without help. She introduced her two visiting daughters to the assessor by name. She also provided a brief social history. This information was validated as accurate via a conversation with her daughters, a review of the hospital discharge summary, and a review of the labels on the medication bottles.
>
> **For Item C2a, Mrs. L should receive a score of "0" for "Yes, memory OK".**
>
> **For Item C2b, she should receive a score of "0" for "Yes, memory OK".**
>
> **For Item C2c, she should receive a score of "0" for "Yes, memory OK".**

Section C Cognition

> Mr. I is a 63-year-old divorced gentleman with a 30-year history of alcohol abuse. Three weeks prior to intake into the home care program, Mr. I passed out while smoking in bed in his rented room, sustaining second-degree burns on his left ear, neck, and chest. He was admitted to an acute care hospital for treatment of burns, smoke inhalation, and delirium tremens. During the first few days of hospitalization he was resuscitated after a respiratory arrest and placed on mechanical ventilation for 5 days. He was transferred to a nursing facility 13 days ago and spent 10 days in a recuperative state.
>
> During the admission assessment to the home care program, which occurred 2 days after his discharge from the nursing home, Mr. I was able to recall the fire but was sketchy on the details of his hospitalization and treatment. He was unable to recall any of the three items posed to him during a test of his short-term memory. Mr. I did relay information about his early life, including his 10-year marriage, the names of his three sons from whom he is now estranged, and his prior work as an accountant (information validated as accurate from his medical record). Mr. I has been able to recognize the faces of his homemakers and of those providing care to him in the home and knows their roles (the nurse and the "therapist"). He also can find his way from his home, can remember his rehabilitation and medical schedules, and prepares and eats lunch with no help from others.
>
> **For Item C2a, Mr. I should receive a score of "1" for "Memory problem".**
>
> **For Item C2b, he should receive a score of "0" for "Yes, memory OK".**
>
> **For Item C2c, he should receive a score of "0" for "Yes, memory OK".**

C3. Periodic Disordered Thinking or Awareness

Intent   To record behavioral signs that may indicate that delirium is present. Frequently, delirium (an acute confusional state) is caused by a treatable illness such as an infection or a reaction to medications.

The characteristics of delirium are often manifested behaviorally and therefore can be observed. For example, disordered thinking may result in rambling, irrelevant, or incoherent speech.

A recent and perhaps rapid deterioration in cognitive function is likely indicative of delirium, which may be reversible if detected and treated in a timely fashion. Signs of delirium can be easier to detect in a person with intact cognitive function at baseline. When a person has a pre-existing cognitive impairment or pre-existing behaviors such as restlessness, calling out, etc., detecting signs of delirium is more difficult. Despite this difficulty, it is possible to detect signs of delirium by being attuned to recent changes in the person's usual functioning. For example, a person who is usually noisy or belligerent may suddenly become quiet, lethargic, and inattentive. Conversely, one who is normally quiet and content may suddenly become restless and noisy.

Definitions

C3a. **Easily distracted** — For example, episodes of difficulty paying attention; person gets sidetracked.

C3b. **Episodes of disorganized speech** — For example, speech is nonsensical, irrelevant, or rambling from subject to subject; person loses train of thought.

C3c. **Mental function varies over the course of the day** — Sometimes better, sometimes worse; behaviors sometimes present, sometimes not.

Process   Ask the person or others who know the person if any of the behaviors have been

	noticed over the last 3 days. If the response is yes, determine whether the behavior is different from the person's normal functioning.
Coding	Code for the person's behavior in the last 3 days regardless of what you believe the cause to be, focusing on when the manifested behavior first occurred and whether it is different from the person's usual pattern.

0. **Behavior not present**
1. **Behavior present, consistent with usual functioning**
2. **Behavior present, appears different from usual functioning** — for example, new onset or worsening, different from a few weeks ago. |

Examples of How to Code Indicators of Periodic Disordered Thinking or Awareness

Tom was observed to have episodes of rambling speech on 2 of the last 3 days. This behavior has been present for some time and has not changed in approximate frequency. It occurs during the day and evening; Tom generally sleeps through the night. He is able to attend to conversations with his caregiver, however.

- Item C3a should be scored "0" for "Behavior not present".
- Item C3b should be scored "1" for "Behavior present, consistent with usual functioning".
- Item C3c should be scored "0" for "Behavior not present".

Mr. Smith has been observed to be picking at his clothing when he is spoken to and rambles incoherently whenever he is awake. These are new behaviors, according to his family.

- Item C3a should be scored "2" for "Behavior present, appears different from usual functioning".
- Item C3b should be scored "2" for "Behavior present, appears different from usual functioning".
- Item C3c should be scored "0" for "Behavior not present".

C4.	**Acute Change in Mental Status from Person's Usual Functioning**
Definition	Any sudden or recent change in the person's usual level of functioning; such changes may include restlessness, lethargy, being difficult to arouse, or altered environmental perception.
Coding	0. No
1. Yes

C5.	**Change in Decision Making as Compared to 90 Days Ago (or Since Last Assessment if Less Than 90 Days Ago)**
Intent	To compare the person's current decision-making ability to that of 90 days ago (or since the last assessment, if that was less than 90 days ago). The changes may be

permanent or temporary, and the cause may be known (for example, psychotropic medication or new pain) or unknown. If the person is newly admitted to the program, include changes since admission **and** changes during the period prior to admission.

Process Talk to the person and family members. Ask them to compare the person's decision-making status now versus 90 days ago (or since the last assessment if less than 90 days ago). To help identify the 90-day time period, ask the person or others to pinpoint an event that occurred 3 months ago, and then to relate the person's functioning to that event. For example, if the person visited a family member 3 months ago, ask how able he or she was in making decisions during that trip.

Coding
0. Improved
1. No change
2. Declined
8. Uncertain

Section D

Communication and Vision

D1. Making Self Understood (Expression)

Intent To document the person's ability to express or communicate requests, needs, opinions, and urgent problems and to engage in social conversation. Such communication may take the form of speech, writing, sign language, or a combination of these (includes use of word board or keyboard).

Process Interact with the person. Observe and listen to the person's efforts to communicate with you. If possible, observe his or her interactions with family. If he or she has communication devices, encourage their use during the assessment. Observe the person's interactions with others in different settings (for example, one-on-one, in groups, with family members) and different circumstances (for example, when calm, when agitated). Note that this item is not intended to address differences in language understanding, such as only speaking in a language not familiar to the assessor.

Coding Enter the number corresponding to the most correct response.

  0. **Understood** — The person expresses ideas clearly without difficulty.
  1. **Usually understood** — The person has difficulty finding the right words or finishing thoughts (resulting in delayed responses), **but** if given time, requires little or no prompting.
  2. **Often understood** — The person has difficulty finding words or finishing thoughts, and prompting is usually required.
  3. **Sometimes understood** — The person has limited ability, but is able to express **concrete** requests regarding at least basic needs (such as food, drink, sleep, toilet).
  4. **Rarely or never understood** — At best, understanding is limited to interpretation of highly individual, person-specific sounds or body language (for example, caregiver has learned to interpret person signaling the presence of pain or need to toilet).

D2. Ability to Understand Others (Comprehension)

Intent To describe the person's ability to comprehend verbal information, whether communicated to the person orally, in writing, or through sign language or Braille. This item measures the person's ability not only to hear messages but also to process and understand language.

Process Interact with the person. Consult with family.

Coding Enter the number corresponding to the most correct response.

0. Understands — Clearly comprehends the speaker's message(s) and demonstrates comprehension by words or actions/behaviors.

1. Usually understands — With little or no prompting, person misses some part or intent of the message but comprehends most of it. The person may have periodic difficulties integrating information but generally demonstrates comprehension by responding in words or actions.

2. Often understands — The person misses some part or intent of the message. However, with prompting (repetition or more detailed explanation), the person often comprehends the conversation.

3. Sometimes understands — The person demonstrates frequent difficulties integrating information, and responds adequately only to simple and direct questions or directions. When the message is rephrased or simplified, or gestures are used, the person's comprehension is enhanced.

4. Rarely or never understands — The person demonstrates very limited ability to understand communication, or the assessor cannot determine whether the person comprehends messages, based on his or her verbal and nonverbal responses. Includes situations where the person can hear sounds but does not understand messages.

D3. Hearing

Intent

To evaluate the person's ability to hear (with environmental adjustments, if necessary) during the past 3-day period.

Process

Evaluate hearing ability after the person has a hearing appliance in place (if the person uses an appliance). Be sure to ask if the battery works and the hearing aid is on. Interview and observe the person, and ask about hearing function. Consult the person's family. Test the accuracy of your findings by observing the person during your verbal interactions.

Ask the person about hearing function, and observe for hearing function during your verbal interactions. Use a variety of observations to make your assessment (for example, one-on-one vs. in group situations). If possible, observe the person interacting with others (such as family members). Always be mindful of environmental factors (nearby conversations, outside noises, etc.) that could influence your assessment. If necessary, consult with the family, primary support people, or speech or hearing specialists to clarify the person's exact hearing level.

Be alert to what you have to do to communicate with the person. Clues that there is a hearing problem include having to speak more clearly or slowly, or use a louder tone or more gestures. Persons with hearing problems may also need to see your face to know what you are saying, or you may have to take the person to a more quiet area to conduct the interview.

Also, if possible, observe the person interacting with others.

Coding

Enter the number corresponding to the most correct response.

0. Adequate — No difficulty in normal conversation, social interaction, listening to TV.

1. Minimal difficulty — Difficulty in some environments (for example, when the other person speaks softly or is more than 6 feet [2 meters] away).

2. Moderate difficulty — Problem hearing normal conversation, requires quiet setting to hear well.

3. Severe difficulty — Difficulty in all situations (for example, speaker has to talk loudly or speak very slowly, or person reports that all speech is mumbled).

4. No hearing

D4. Vision

Intent

To evaluate the person's ability to see close objects in adequate light, using the person's customary visual appliances for close vision (such as glasses or a magnifying glass).

Definition

Adequate light — What is sufficient or comfortable for a person with normal vision.

Process

Ask person, family member, or home care staff if the person has manifested any change in usual vision patterns over the past 3 days—for example, is the person still able to read newsprint, greeting cards, and the like?

Ask the person about his or her visual abilities. Test the accuracy of your findings by asking the person to look at regular-size print in a book or newspaper with whatever visual appliance he or she customarily uses for close vision (such as glasses or a magnifying glass). Then ask the person to read aloud, starting with larger headlines and ending with the finest, smallest print.

Be sensitive to the fact that some persons are not literate or are unable to read English. In such cases, ask the person to read aloud individual letters or numbers (such as dates or page numbers), or to name items in small pictures.

If the person is unable to communicate or follow your directions for testing vision, observe the person's eye movements to see if his or her eyes seem to follow movement and objects. Though these are gross measurements of visual acuity, they may assist you in assessing whether the person has any visual ability.

Coding

Enter the number corresponding to the most correct response.

0. Adequate — The person sees fine detail, including regular print in newspapers/books.

1. Minimal difficulty — The person sees large print, but not regular print in newspapers/books.

2. Moderate difficulty — The person has limited vision; is not able to see newspaper headlines, but can identify objects in his or her environment.

3. Severe difficulty — The person's ability to identify objects in his or her environment is in question, but the person's eye movements appear to be following objects (especially people walking by). Also includes the ability to see only light, colors, or shapes.

NOTE: Many persons with severe cognitive impairment are unable to participate in vision screening because they are unable to follow directions or are unable to tell you what they see. However, many such persons appear to "track" or follow moving objects in their environment with their eyes. For persons who appear to do this, score the item **"3"** for "Severe difficulty". This is often the best assessment you can do with the limited technology available in the home care environment.

4. No vision — The person has no vision; eyes do not appear to be following objects (especially people walking by).

Section E

Mood and Behavior

Mood distress is a serious condition and is associated with significant morbidity. Associated factors include poor adjustment to one's living situation, functional impairment, resistance to daily care, inability to participate in activities, social isolation, increased risk of medical illness, cognitive impairment, and an increased sensitivity to physical pain. It is particularly important to identify signs and symptoms of mood distress because they are treatable.

It would be very unusual for family members to have received specific training in how to evaluate persons who have distressed mood or behavioral symptoms. Therefore, although family may sense that something is wrong, mood distress is often underdiagnosed and undertreated in community settings. Thus, this assessment may serve as a crucial first opportunity to identify whether such problems are present.

E1. Indicators of Possible Depressed, Anxious, or Sad Mood

Intent To record the presence of indicators observed in the last 3 days, irrespective of the assumed cause of the indicator/behavior.

Definitions The mental state indicators may be expressed verbally through direct statements or through nonverbal indicators or behaviors that can be monitored by observing the person during usual daily routines.

- **E1a. Made negative statements** — For example, "Nothing matters"; "Would rather be dead than live this way"; "What's the use"; "Regret having lived so long"; "Let me die."

- **E1b. Persistent anger with self or others** — For example, easily annoyed, anger at care received.

- **E1c. Expressions, including nonverbal, of what appear to be unrealistic fears** — For example, fear of being abandoned, being left alone, or being with others; intense fear of specific objects or situations.

- **E1d. Repetitive health complaints** — For example, persistently seeks medical attention, incessant concern with body functions.

- **E1e. Repetitive anxious complaints/concerns (non-health-related)** — For example, persistently seeks attention/reassurance regarding schedules, meals, laundry, clothing, and relationships.

- **E1f. Sad, pained, or worried facial expressions** — For example, furrowed brows, constant frowning.

- **E1g. Crying, tearfulness** — Distress may also be expressed through such nonverbal indications.

- **E1h. Recurrent statements that something terrible is about to happen** — For example, believes he or she is about to die, have a heart attack.

- **E1i. Withdrawal from activities of interest** — Including long-standing activities, being with family/friends.

E1j. Reduced social interactions

E1k. Expressions, including nonverbal, of a lack of pleasure in life (anhedonia)
— For example, saying "I don't enjoy anything anymore."

Process

Feelings of psychic distress may be expressed directly by the person who is depressed, anxious, or sad. Distress can also be expressed through nonverbal indicators. Initiate a conversation with the person, being cognizant of earlier statements by (or observations of) the person. Some persons are more verbal about their feelings than others and will either tell someone about their distress, or will at least tell someone when asked directly how they feel. For persons who verbalize their feelings, ask how long these conditions have been present. Other persons may be unable to articulate their feelings (perhaps because they cannot find the words to describe how they feel, or lack insight or cognitive capacity). Observe the person carefully for any indicator, both at the time of the planned assessment and in any direct contacts you may have with the person during the 3 days covered by this assessment. Consult with family members who have direct knowledge of the person's typical and current behavior, and any other clinicians working with the person (such as the primary care provider, if available).

Remember to be aware of cultural differences in how these indicators may be manifested. Some persons may be more or less expressive of mental health concerns, emotions, or feelings because of their cultural norms. Be cautious not to minimize your interpretation of an indicator based on your expectations about the person's cultural background. On the other hand, it is important to be especially sensitive to these indicators when assessing a person whose culture may make him or her more stoic in his or her expressions.

Coding

Based on your interaction with and observation of the person, score each indicator based on the person's behavior over the last 3 days using one of the following codes. Remember, score each item based on what you see or what is reported to you, regardless of what you believe the cause to be.

0. Not present

1. Present but not exhibited in last 3 days — Use this code if you know the condition is present and active, even though it was not observed over the last 3 days.

2. Exhibited on 1–2 of last 3 days

3. Exhibited daily in last 3 days

E2. Self-Reported Mood

Intent

To record the person's self-reported mood over the last 3 days. In some cases, the person may deny feeling a particular way in the last 3 days, but reports that the issue continues to be "present" and active.

Definitions

These items involve verbal reports of the person's subjective evaluation of three dimensions of mood state (i.e., anhedonia, anxiety, dysphoria) over the last 3 days.

"In the last 3 days, how often have you felt . . .?"

E2a. Little interest or pleasure in things you normally enjoy?

E2b. Anxious, restless, or uneasy?

E2c. Sad, depressed, or hopeless?

Process	Ask the person the previous questions directly once you have completed your own ratings of the person's mood state using the other items in the Mood section of the assessment. **Only the person's responses** should be used to rate each item. Do not code the items based on your own inferences about the person's mood state and do not record ratings given by family, friends, or other informants. These items should be treated strictly as self-report measures. If the person is unable (due to cognitive impairment, for example) or refuses to respond, do not dwell on these items and do not impute responses for the person. Use code "8" in such a situation.
Coding	Code each item using the **person's response as to whether/how often he or she experienced the feelings referenced in the items** over the last 3 days, regardless of what the person believes to be the underlying cause of these feelings. Remember to code for both the presence of the indicator and the number of days in which it was felt, no matter how often it was felt per day. Persons unable or unwilling to respond should be scored "8" for "Person could not (would not) respond". Use the following codes:

0. **Not in last 3 days**

1. **Not in last 3 days, but often feels that way** — Use this code only if the person indicates the feeling is frequently **present** and **active**, but was not experienced in the last 3 days.

2. **In 1–2 of last 3 days**

3. **Daily in the last 3 days**

8. **Person could not (would not) respond**

E3. Behavior Symptoms

Intent	To identify the frequency of behavioral symptoms during the last 3 days that cause distress to the person, or are distressing or disruptive to others with whom the person lives. Such behaviors include those that are potentially harmful to the person or disruptive to others. These items are designed to pick up problem behaviors exhibited by the person that may be considered as "combative or agitated" by some health professionals. Acknowledging and documenting behavioral symptoms provides a basis for further evaluation, care planning, and delivery of consistent, appropriate care toward ameliorating the behavioral symptoms.
Definitions	E3a. **Wandering** — Moved about with no discernible, rational purpose. A wandering person may be oblivious to his or her physical or safety needs. Wandering behavior should be differentiated from purposeful movement (such as a hungry person moving about the apartment in search of food). Wandering may be by walking or by wheelchair. Do not include pacing back and forth, which is not considered wandering.
	E3b. **Verbal abuse** — For example, others were threatened, screamed at, or cursed at.
	E3c. **Physical abuse** — For example, others were hit, shoved, scratched, or sexually abused.
	E3d. **Socially inappropriate or disruptive behavior** — For example, made disruptive sounds or noises, screamed out, smeared or threw food or feces, hoarded, or rummaged through others' belongings.
	E3e. **Inappropriate public sexual behavior or public disrobing**

E3f. Resists care — For example, resisted taking medications/injections; pushed caregiver while receiving assistance with ADLs, eating, or changing position. This category does not include instances where the person has made an informed choice not to follow a course of care (for example, the person has exercised his or her right to refuse treatment, and reacts negatively as others try to reinstitute treatment). Signs of resistance may be verbal or physical (such as verbally refusing care, pushing caregiver away, scratching caregiver). These behaviors are not necessarily positive or negative; the item is intended to provide information about the person's responses to interventions and to prompt further investigation of causes for care planning purposes. Such causes might include fear of pain, fear of falling, poor comprehension, anger, poor relationships, eagerness for greater participation in care decisions, past experience with medication errors and unacceptable care, or desire to modify the care being provided.

Process

Ask the family member or caregiver if each specified problem behavior occurred. Take an objective view of the person's behavioral symptoms, and focus on the person's actions, not intent. It is often difficult to determine the meaning behind a particular behavioral symptom. The fact that some family members have become used to the behavior or minimize the person's presumed intent ("He doesn't really mean to hurt anyone—he's just frightened") should not be considered in coding items. Rather, code each item based on whether the person manifested the behavioral symptom.

Observe the person and the way he or she responds to attempts by family members or others to deliver care. Ask caregivers if they know what occurred throughout the day and night for the past 3 days. If possible, try to do this when the person is not in the room. Recognize that responses given with the person present may need to be validated later. Also, the presence of multiple caregivers during the assessment may discourage individuals from answering accurately.

Coding

0. Not present

1. Present but not exhibited in last 3 days — This code indicates that while the assessor knows the condition is present and active, it was not physically manifested over the last 3 days.

2. Exhibited on 1–2 of last 3 days

3. Exhibited daily in last 3 days

Examples of How to Code Behavior Symptoms

Mr. W has dementia and is severely impaired in making daily decisions. He wanders all around the apartment throughout the day. He is extremely hard of hearing and refuses to wear his hearing aid. He is easily frightened by others and cannot stay still when anyone visits. Numerous attempts more than a week ago to redirect his wandering resulted in his hitting and pushing family. Over time, family members have found him to be most content while he is wandering within the structured setting of the apartment. **Code as follows:**

Item E3a ("Wandering") should be scored "3" for "Exhibited daily in last 3 days".

Item E3b ("Verbal abuse") should be scored "0" for "Not present".

Item E3c ("Physical abuse") should be scored "1" for "Present but not exhibited in last 3 days".

Item E3d ("Socially inappropriate or disruptive behavior") should be scored "0" for "Not present".

Item E3e ("Inappropriate public sexual behavior or disrobing") should be scored "0" for "Not present".

Item E3f ("Resists care") should be scored "0" for "Not present".

Mrs. N's daughter states she has found her mother going through the daughter's closet in the middle of the night. This has happened on 2 of the last 3 nights. When she tried to get her mother to return to her own room and bed, the mother became angry and shouted at her daughter. She accused the daughter of stealing her things. **Code as follows:**

Item E3a ("Wandering") should be scored "0" for "Not present".

Item E3b ("Verbal abuse") should be scored "2" for "Exhibited on 1–2 of last 3 days".

Item E3c ("Physical abuse") should be scored "0" for "Not present".

Item E3d ("Socially inappropriate or disruptive behavior") should be scored "2" for "Exhibited on 1–2 of last 3 days".

Item E3e ("Inappropriate public sexual behavior or disrobing") should be scored "0" for "Not present".

Item E3f ("Resists care") should be scored "0" for "Not present".

Section F

Psychosocial Well-Being

F1. Social Relationships

Intent To document and describe the person's interaction patterns and adaptation to his or her social environment. To assess the degree to which the person is involved in social activities, meaningful roles, and daily pursuits.

Definitions

F1a. Participation in social activities of long-standing interest — The person engaged in social activities that have been of long-standing interest to him or her. The activities may be quite varied and should be counted as long as they involve interaction with at least one other person. Examples include attending meetings of informal clubs or religious services, playing bridge or bingo, volunteering at the local clothing bank, or gossiping with the neighbors on their front porches in the evening.

F1b. Visit with a long-standing social relation or family member — The person was visited by (or made a visit to) any family member, friend, or social acquaintance with a long-standing relationship with the person (for example, a neighbor or fellow member of a community organization or religious group). The focus here is on well-established, informal ties rather than visits with paid staff, volunteers, or new acquaintances.

F1c. Other interaction with long-standing social relation or family member — For example, telephone or e-mail. The person interacted through a means other than a face-to-face visit with a family member, friend, or social acquaintance with a long-standing relationship with the person (such as a neighbor or fellow member of a community organization or religious group). As with Item F1b, the focus is on well-established, informal ties rather than contacts by paid staff, volunteers, or new acquaintances.

F1d. Conflict or anger with family or friends — The person expresses feelings such as abandonment, ingratitude on part of the family, lack of understanding by close friends, or hostility regarding relationships with family or friends.

F1e. Fearful of a family member or close acquaintance — The person expresses (verbally or through behavior) fear of a family member or close acquaintance. Such fear can be expressed in many ways. A person may state that he or she is afraid of a caregiver, or may appear to withdraw whenever the caregiver is around. This may include fear of physical or emotional abuse or mistreatment. It is not necessary to establish the reason for the fear, only to determine whether it is present.

F1f. Neglected, abused, or mistreated — The person experienced a serious or life-threatening situation or condition that went untreated or was not appropriately acknowledged. The situation may have put the person at risk of death, or of complications that impinge on physical or mental health.

Process Ask the person for his or her point of view. What activities does he or she enjoy participating in? When was the last time he or she was able to participate? Who tends to come to visit, and when was the last time that individual visited? Are there other ways the person contacts family or friends (for example, by telephone or e-mail)? Is the person generally content or unhappy in relationships with family and friends? If the person is unhappy, what specifically is he or she unhappy about?

If possible, also talk with family members and friends who visit or have frequent telephone contact with the person. The primary caregiver may have a good sense of who visits or contacts the person. He or she can also describe the most common social activities the person was involved in recently.

Coding	0. Never
	1. More than 30 days ago
	2. 8 to 30 days ago
	3. 4 to 7 days ago
	4. In last 3 days
	8. Unable to determine

NOTE: Score "8" for "Unable to determine" if no information is available from the person or other informants about the person's social relationships.

Example of How to Code for Conflict or Anger with Family or Friends

Mr. H tells the assessor he has to do what his daughter says or "she gets mad with me." He said that he sees her every weekend and she "bosses" him around. When the assessor talks to his daughter, she reports no conflict. The assessment takes place on a Thursday.

Code as "3" (Yes, openly expresses conflict 4 to 7 days ago).

F2.	**Lonely**
Definition	The person states or otherwise indicates that he or she feels lonely. The person may feel that others do not visit enough or desire more social interaction even if visited regularly. Others may also report that the person sometimes comments on feeling lonely.
Process	Talk with the person to determine whether or not he or she feels lonely. If possible, speak with the person's family or other informal contacts (such as neighbors) to get their perception of the person's feelings of loneliness.
Coding	0. No
	1. Yes
F3.	**Change in Social Activities in Last 90 Days (or Since Last Assessment if Less Than 90 Days Ago)**
Intent	To identify a recent change (as compared to 90 days ago—or since the last assessment, if less than 90 days have passed) in the person's level of participation in social, religious, occupational, or other preferred activities. If the level of participation has declined, determine whether the person is distressed by it.
Definition	The level of participation refers to the quantity (how many) of different types of

social activities; the intensity (how frequently contact occurs); and the quality of the activity (how deeply the person is involved). Remote participation is equally important and significant for the person's role fulfillment and self-esteem (for example, a person who cannot move outside his or her home may still participate or be associated with some kind of religious, political, or social activity). Distress occurs when the person's mood is adversely affected by a recent change in the level of participation (as evidenced by sadness, loss of motivation or self-esteem, anxiety, or depression, for example).

Process	Talk with the person to determine whether a change has occurred and to determine his or her subjective response to any changes. If possible, speak with the family or other informal contacts (such as neighbors) to get their opinions on whether the person's activity levels have changed and, if so, how he or she responded to those changes.
Coding	0. **No decline** — There was no change or there was an increase in the person's level of participation in social activities.
	1. **Decline, not distressed** — The person experienced a decline in his or her level of participation in social activities without a corresponding increase in his or her distress.
	2. **Decline, distressed** — Both decline and distress are observed or reported.

F4. Length of Time Alone During the Day (Morning and Afternoon)

Intent	To identify the actual amount of time the person is alone.
Definition	The amount of time the person is literally alone, without any other person in the home. If the person is residing in a board and care facility, congregate housing, or other situation where there are other persons in their own rooms, count the amount of time the person spends by him- or herself in the person's own room as time alone.
Process	First ask the person how much time he or she spends alone. Be clear about how "being alone" is defined. Confirm with caregivers the amount of time the person spends alone.
Coding	Code for the most appropriate category.
	0. Less than 1 hour
	1. 1–2 hours
	2. More than 2 hours but less than 8 hours
	3. 8 hours or more

F5. Major Life Stressors in Last 90 Days

Intent	To identify any life events that the person considers to have had a major impact on his or her life in the last 90 days.
Definition	**Life stressors** — Experiences that either disrupted or threatened to disrupt a person's daily routine and that imposed some degree of readjustment.

Process	Ask the person if any stressful events have occurred in the last 90 days. Examples may include an episode of severe personal illness, the death or severe illness of a close family member or friend, the loss of the person's home, a major loss of income or assets, being the victim of a crime such as robbery or assault, the loss of the person's driving license or car, etc.
Coding	**0. No** **1. Yes**

Section G

Functional Status

G1.	**IADL Self-Performance and Capacity**
Intent	To examine the areas of function that are most commonly associated with independent living (instrumental activities of daily living, or IADLs).
Definitions	**G1a. Meal preparation** — How meals are prepared (planning meals, assembling ingredients, cooking, setting out food and utensils). This item should be assessed in terms of the person's ability to put meals together, regardless of the quality or nutritional value of the meal. For example, if the person is able to make cold cereal for breakfast, or put together a cold sandwich and drink coffee at lunch, or make toast for dinner without assistance, the person would be scored as independent in meal preparation capacity.
	G1b. Ordinary housework — How ordinary work around the house is performed (for example, doing dishes, dusting, making bed, tidying up, laundry).
	G1c. Managing finances — How bills are paid, checkbook is balanced, household expenses are budgeted, and credit card account is monitored.
	G1d. Managing medications — How medications are managed (for example, remembering to take medicines, opening bottles, taking correct drug dosages, giving injections, applying ointments).
	G1e. Phone use — How telephone calls are made or received (with assistive devices such as large numbers on telephone, amplification as needed).
	G1f. Stairs — How a **full** flight of stairs is managed (i.e., 12–14 stairs). If the person is able to go up and down only a half flight (2–6 stairs), do not score as independent.
	G1g. Shopping — How shopping is performed for food and household items (selecting items, paying money). **This item does not include transportation.**
	G1h. Transportation — How person travels by public transportation (navigating system, paying fare) or drives self (including getting out of the house, into and out of vehicles).
Process	Question the person about his or her performance of normal activities around the home or in the community in the last 3 days. You may also talk to family members if they are available. Use your own observations as you are gathering information for other interRAI HC Assessment items.
Coding	Each item should be scored in two categories: Performance and Capacity.
	Performance — Measures what the person actually did within each IADL category in the last 3 days. Do not base your coding on what the person might be capable of doing (see the Capacity category).
	Capacity — Code based on the person's presumed ability to carry out the activity. This requires speculation by the assessor.

Because of lack of skills or experience, a person may not perform some activities, but would be capable of doing so with the proper training or opportunity. Therefore, it is important to distinguish between nonperformance that is due to impairment of capability (caused by health problems) and nonperformance that is due to other factors (not related to the person's health). For example, some males may never have learned to cook, and some females may never have handled financial matters. For some activities, the person may perform the activity independently at times, but receive/require assistance at other times. First, determine whether the person actually performed the activity. If not, evaluate whether the person is capable of performing the task.

0. **Independent** — No help, setup, or supervision needed.
1. **Setup help only**
2. **Supervision** — Oversight/cuing required.
3. **Limited assistance** — Help required on some occasions.
4. **Extensive assistance** — Help required throughout task, but performs 50% or more of task on own.
5. **Maximal assistance** — Help required throughout task, but performs less than 50% of task on own.
6. **Total dependence** — Full performance of activity during entire period by others.
8. **Activity did not occur** — During entire period. **NOTE: You may use this code to score the Performance category, but do not use it to score Capacity category.**

Examples of How to Code IADLs

Mrs. Q does not do her own shopping. Her daughter visits every Sunday, gets the list from her mother, and does the shopping. While appreciating her daughter's help, Mrs. Q feels she would have no difficulty doing the shopping herself. **In the Performance category, Item G1g should be scored "6" for "Total dependence". In the Capacity category, Item G1g should be scored "0" for "Independent".**

The following is a possible conversation between the assessor and a person regarding Item G1a, "Meal preparation".

Assessor: Do you prepare your own meals? For example, do you plan your meals, gather ingredients together, cook, and lay out your food utensils?

Person: *No, I can't do it.*

Assessor: Who gets your breakfast?

Person: *I get myself some cold cereal.*

Assessor: How about lunch?

Person: *I get meals-on-wheels 5 days a week.*

Assessor: What about the weekends?

Person: *They leave me enough to heat up in the microwave—or my neighbors or family send lunch over.*

Assessor: Who fixes dinner?

Person: *I just fix a snack, or my homemaker fixes dinner and leaves it to be heated up.*

Assessor: Could you manage to get yourself something to eat without this help?

Person: *All I could do is get some cold food. I am really too unsteady to cook at a stove.*

In the Performance category, Item G1a should be scored "5" for "Maximal assistance". In the Capacity category, Item G1a should be scored "4" for "Extensive assistance".

Here is another sample conversation regarding meals.

Assessor: Do you prepare your own meals?
Person: *No, my wife takes care of that.*
Assessor: Do you ever get your own breakfast?
Person: *No, she gets me cold cereal and fruit with coffee every morning.*
Assessor: Do you ever get your own lunch?
Person: *Sometimes if my wife is out.*
Assessor: Did you do it in the last 3 days?
Person: *No.*
Assessor: So, are you saying that she prepares the main meal and heavy cooking?
Person: *Yes.*
Assessor: Could you do the cooking if you had to?
Person: *Yes—not as well as my wife, as she is a real pro, but I could manage.*

In the Performance category, Item G1a should be scored "6" for "Total dependence".
In the Capacity category, Item G1a should be scored "0" for "Independent".

Additional Examples of How to Code IADLs

IADL	Performance Category	Capacity Category
Mrs. Y has not made any meals for herself over the last 3 days. Her daughter is visiting and she is doing all the cooking. Mrs. Y tells you she can do all her own meal preparation.	For the last 3 days Mrs. Y's daughter has been making the meals. **Code = 6, Total dependence**	Client states she usually fixes her own meals. **Code = 0, Independent**
Mr. D's niece helps him with finances such as paying bills and keeping track of the accounts. Mr. D and his niece work on this together. Mr. D gets the bills out and the checkbook and bank accounts. The niece writes out the checks, puts stamps on envelopes, and mails them. She also does any needed banking. Mr. D likes this arrangement and feels that he would be unable to do any more of the activity himself. Over the last 3 days, Mr. D has not done any financial activities.	In the last 3 days, Mr. D has not done any financial management. **In this category, Item G1c should be scored "8" for "Activity did not occur".**	Mr. D's niece helps him with finances. She does more than 50% of the subtasks. **In this category, Item G1c should be scored "5" for "Maximal Assistance".**
Ms. A has a visit from a skilled nurse every week. The nurse puts 7 days' worth of correct medications into Ms. A's pill caddy. The nurse calls in the refills and the pharmacy delivers them. Ms. A does remember to take her medications each day on her own. The nurse refilled her pill caddy 3 days ago. Ms. A has problems with remembering to take her medications correctly if the prefilled caddy is not available.	All Ms. A does by herself is remembering to take pills in the caddy and swallowing them at the correct times. The nurse is doing more than 50% of subtasks of medication management. **In this category, Item G1d should be scored "5" for "Maximal Assistance".**	There is no difference between Ms. D's performance and capacity. **In this category, Item G1d should also be scored "5" for "Maximal Assistance".**

Section G Functional Status

G2. ADL Self-Performance

Intent To record what the person did for him- or herself and how others assisted in the performance of self-care activities of daily living (ADLs) during the last 3 days.

Definitions **ADL self-performance** — Measures based on all episodes of the activity over the last 3 days. The following are the performance-based items.

> **G2a. Bathing** — How the person takes a full-body bath or shower. Includes how person transfers in and out of tub or shower and how each part of body is bathed: arms, upper and lower legs, chest, abdomen and perineal area. **EXCLUDE WASHING OF BACK AND HAIR.**
>
> **G2b. Personal hygiene** — How the person manages personal hygiene, including combing hair, brushing teeth, shaving, applying make-up, washing and drying face and hands. **EXCLUDE BATHS AND SHOWERS.**
>
> **G2c. Dressing upper body** — How the person dresses and undresses (street clothes, underwear) above the waist, including prostheses, orthotics, fasteners, pullovers, etc.
>
> **G2d. Dressing lower body** — How the person dresses and undresses (street clothes, underwear) from the waist down, including prostheses, orthotics, belts, pants, skirt, shoes, fasteners, etc.
>
> **G2e. Walking** — How the person walks between locations on the same floor indoors.
>
> **G2f. Locomotion** — How the person moves between locations on the same floor (walking or wheeling). If the person uses a wheelchair, this measures self-sufficiency once he or she is in the chair.
>
> **G2g. Transfer toilet** — How the person moves on and off the toilet or commode.
>
> **G2h. Toilet use** — How the person uses the toilet room (or commode, bedpan, urinal), cleanses him- or herself after toilet use or incontinent episode(s), changes bed pad, manages ostomy or catheter, adjusts clothes. **This item does not include transfer on and off the toilet.**
>
> **G2i. Bed mobility** — How the person moves to and from a lying position, turns from side to side, and positions his or her body while in bed.
>
> **G2j. Eating** — How the person eats and drinks (regardless of skill). Includes intake of nourishment by other means (such as tube feeding or total parenteral nutrition).
>
> **Setup help** — Assistance characterized by the provision of articles, devices, or preparation necessary for the person's self-performance of an activity. This includes giving or holding out an item the person takes from the helper, if the helper then leaves the person alone to complete the activity. If someone remains nearby to watch over the person, the person is receiving oversight, thus the score would be **"2"** for "Supervision". Following are a few examples of setup help. For the "Personal hygiene" item, setup help might mean providing a washbasin or grooming articles. For "Walking", it might take the form of handing the person a walker or cane. For "Toilet use", it might be handing the person a bedpan or placing within reach the articles necessary for changing an ostomy appliance. For "Eating", setup help might include cutting meat or opening containers at meals, carrying a tray to the table, or giving one food category at a time.

Weight bearing — Persons require varying degrees of physical assistance to complete ADL tasks. A key concept in scoring the degree of assistance is the degree of weight-bearing support provided. When relating to non-upright positions, such support might take the form of a helper holding the full weight of an arm while assisting the person with putting on a shirt. When relating to standing or walking, such support might mean taking the person's weight by holding him or her under the armpit, or allowing the person to lean on the helper's arm. Guiding movements with minimal physical contact and contact guarding with intermittent physical assistance are **not** considered weight bearing.

Process

To describe functioning, the assessor should first get a sense of the episodes in each ADL area over the last 3 days. Determine what the person does for him- or herself and the nature of assistance provided (if any).

When ADL self-performance in an area varies over the last 3 days, identify the three most dependent episodes—i.e., the episodes when the person received the greatest care or assistance from others. The summarization that is done to develop the ADL scores (as described below) focuses on the most dependent episodes, providing a picture of the person's need for help from others in managing the ADLs.

In order to summarize ADL self-performance, gather information as follows:

Gather information from multiple sources. For example, talk with the person, family, staff, and others.

Ask questions pertaining to all aspects of the ADL definitions. For example, when discussing "Personal hygiene" (Item G2b), inquire how the person manages washing in the morning, combing hair, brushing teeth, and shaving. A person can be independent in one aspect of personal hygiene yet require extensive assistance in another aspect.

Observe how the person is performing the physical tasks.

Talk with the person to ascertain what he or she does for him- or herself in each ADL, as well as the type and level of assistance provided by others.

If possible, talk with immediate caregivers or family members.

Finally, weigh all responses to come up with a consistent picture of the person's ADL performance for each episode assessed in each area.

Coding

The following are the ADL Self-Performance scoring rules.

- If **all** episodes in the last 3 days were performed at the same support level, score the ADL at that level.
  - Note that regarding the scores **"0"** ("Independent"), **"6"** ("Total dependence"), and **"8"** ("Activity did not occur"), this is the **only** situation in which such a score would apply. In other words, to receive one of these scores, all performance episodes must be at the same level.
  - Also note that this rule applies when there was only one performance episode during the 3-day period. For example, if over the course of the 3 days the person moved once between locations on the same floor but was bedbound for the remainder of the time, then the score for Item G2f ("Locomotion") should be based on the single episode when the person moved.
- If **any** episodes were at level **"6"** ("Total dependence") and other episodes were less dependent, the item should be scored **"5"** ("Maximal assistance").

- **Otherwise**, focus on the three most dependent episodes (or the two most dependent episodes if the ADL was only performed twice). If the most dependent of these episodes would be scored **"1"** for "Independent, setup help only", score the item **"1"**. If the most dependent of these episodes would receive a higher score, however, the item should receive the score to match the least dependent of those episodes in the range between **"2"** and **"5"**.

In accordance with these rules and the guidelines below, enter the number corresponding to the most correct response.

0. **Independent** — No physical assistance, setup, or supervision in any episode.

1. **Independent, setup help only** — Article or device provided or placed within reach, no physical assistance or supervision in any episode.

2. **Supervision** — Oversight/cuing.

3. **Limited assistance** — Guided maneuvering of limbs, physical guidance without taking weight.

4. **Extensive assistance** — Weight-bearing support (including lifting limbs) by one helper where person still performs 50% or more of subtasks.

5. **Maximal assistance** — Weight-bearing support (including lifting limbs) by two or more helpers; **or**, weight-bearing support for more than 50% of subtasks.

6. **Total dependence** — Full performance by others during all episodes.

8. **Activity did not occur during entire period** — Do not confuse a person's total dependence in an ADL activity (**"6"** for "Total dependence") with nonoccurrence of the activity itself (**"8"**). For example, even a person who receives tube feedings and no food or fluids by mouth is engaged in eating (receiving nourishment) and must be evaluated under the eating category for his or her level of assistance in the process. A person who is highly involved in giving him- or herself a tube feeding is not totally dependent and should not be scored with **"6"**, but with a lower score, dependent on the nature of the help received from others.

Here are general guidelines for recording accurate ADL Self-Performance:

- The coding scale for ADLs records the person's actual level of involvement in self-care and the type and amount of support actually received during the last 3 days.

- Do not base your assessment on the person's capacity for involvement in self-care—i.e., what you believe the person **could** do for him- or herself.

- Do not record the type and level of assistance you think the person "should" be receiving (for example, based on a written plan of care or expectations the family may have). The type and level of assistance actually provided might be quite different from what is indicated in a care plan. Record what is actually happening.

- Engage family (or, when possible, formal home care staff who have cared for the person over the last 3 days) in discussions regarding the person's ADL functions. Remind these persons that the focus is on the last 3 days only. To clarify your own understanding and observations about each ADL activity (bed mobility, walking, transfer toilet, etc.), ask probing questions, beginning with the general and proceeding to the more specific.

G3.	Locomotion/Walking
G3a.	Primary mode of locomotion
Intent	To record the primary mode of locomotion and type of appliances, aids, or assistive devices the person used over the last 3 days.
Definitions	**Cane** — A slender stick held in the hand and used for support when walking.
	Crutch — A device for aiding a person with walking. Usually it is a long staff with a padded crescent-shaped portion at the top that is placed under the armpit.
	Scooter — Motorized vehicle operated by a person for use in getting from one location to another.
	Walker — A mobile device used to assist a person with walking. Usually consists of a stable platform made of metal tubing that the person grasps while taking a step. The person then moves the walker forward and takes another step.
Coding	Code for the primary mode of locomotion used by the person indoors within the last 3 days. For persons who walk by pushing a wheelchair in front of them for support, or by using a walker-type device such as a Merry Walker, use code **"1"** ("Walking, uses assistive device").
	0. Walking, no assistive device
	1. Walking, uses assistive device — For example, a cane, walker, crutch, or pushing wheelchair.
	2. Wheelchair, scooter
	3. Bedbound
G3b.	Timed 13-foot (or 4-meter) walk
Intent	This performance test provides a measure of the person's stamina. It is designed to establish an objective benchmark for comparison with the person's performance upon subsequent reassessments.
Process	Lay out a straight, unobstructed course. Use a tape measure to measure off the 13 feet (4 meters). If possible, mark the beginning and end of the measured distance using nonstaining tape or another device that can be easily removed and will not damage the person's dwelling. You will need to stand very close to the person while he or she is trying to complete the test. Have a chair at hand; if the person becomes weak or is unable to continue, you should have him or her sit on the chair. Say: "When I tell you, begin to walk at a normal pace (with cane/walker if used). This is not a test of how fast you can walk. Stop when I tell you to stop. Is this clear?" You should then demonstrate the test for the person. Have the person stand still, with both feet just touching the starting line. Then say: "Begin to walk now." Start stopwatch (alternately, you can count off seconds out loud—"one one-thousand, two-one-thousand," and so forth) when the person's foot hits the ground with the first step. Stop counting when the person's foot falls beyond the 13-foot (or 4-meter) mark. Then say: "You may stop now."

Coding	This test cannot be done with persons who need any type of physical weight-bearing assistance to walk. For persons who need this type of assistance, use the score **"99"** for "Not tested". If the person is capable of doing the test but chooses not to, enter **"88"** for "Refused to do the test".
For persons who do the test, use the scoring guidelines that follow.
If the person completes the test in less than 30 seconds, enter the number of seconds. (If fewer than 10 seconds, use a leading zero to fill in the first box—for example, **"09"**.)
If the person took 30 or more seconds to complete the test, enter **"30"** as the score.
If the person began the test but did not finish it, enter **"77"** for "Stopped before test complete".
G3c.	**Distance walked**
Intent	To assess the person's independence in walking around the home or the community.
Definition	Farthest distance walked at one time without sitting down in the last 3 days, with support as needed.
Process	Ask the person and family member about the person's walking in the home or community during the last 3 days. Record the farthest distance walked without sitting down.
Coding	**0. Did not walk**
1. Less than 15 feet (under 5 meters)
2. 15–149 feet (5–49 meters)
3. 150–299 feet (50–99 meters)
4. 300+ feet (100+ meters)
5. ½ mile or more (1+ kilometer)
G3d.	**Distance wheeled self**
Intent	To monitor a person's independence in moving about the home or community in a nonmotorized wheelchair (or scooter).
Definition	The farthest distance the person wheeled him- or herself at one time in the last 3 days (includes independent use of motorized wheelchair).
Process	Ask the person and family member about the person's movement in the home or community during the last 3 days. Record the farthest distance traveled without a prolonged stop.
Coding	**0. Wheeled by others**
1. Used motorized wheelchair/scooter
2. Wheeled self less than 15 feet (under 5 meters)
3. Wheeled self 15–149 feet (5–49 meters)
4. Wheeled self 150–299 feet (50–99 meters)
5. Wheeled self 300+ feet (100+ meters)
8. Did not use wheelchair

G4. Activity Level

Intent Moderate physical activity in connection with activities of everyday life or chosen activities can help to keep persons in home care fit in many ways. Below a certain threshold of activity, functional decline may be accelerated.

It is necessary to understand whether the person is motivated to undertake physical activity, what the person's needs may be, what barriers need to be overcome, and whether health education is needed.

Many persons are interested in maintaining health. They usually know that life-style practices may be important, but they often need concrete information about how important their own life-style is for health maintenance. For example, the person may understand the general importance of exercise and good nutrition, but may not be willing or readily able to make changes in his or her life-style without some type of support or assistance.

G4a. Total hours of exercise or physical activity in the LAST 3 DAYS (e.g., walking)

Definition **Exercise or physical activity** — Any exercise that involves at least moderate physical activity, such as walking outdoors, swimming, yoga, class, exercise with machines.

Process Ask the person and family to describe the person's involvement in physical activity in the last 3 days (for example, walking).

Coding If the accumulated time is between 2 hours and 3 hours, use code "2". Hours of exercise do not have to occur all at once on a given day; they may be accumulated over the course of several instances.

0. None
1. Less than 1 hour
2. 1–2 hours
3. 3–4 hours
4. More than 4 hours

G4b. In the LAST 3 DAYS, number of days went out of the house or building in which he/she resides

Definition **Went out of the house or building** — This means the person went outdoors, no matter how short the period of time he or she spent outdoors. This could mean going into the yard, standing on an open porch, or walking down the street.

Process Ask the person or family if the person went outside in the last 3 days.

Coding If illness or weather did not permit (for example, if it snowed or there was a "tropical" downpour) and the person did not leave the house, but normally would have during a 3-day period, use code "1".

0. No days out
1. Did not go out in last 3 days, but usually goes out over a 3-day period
2. 1–2 days
3. 3 days

G5.	**Physical Function Improvement Potential**
Intent	To assess the likelihood that the person has the capacity for greater independence and involvement in his or her care. Item G5a records the person's own opinion; Item G5b records the opinion of a care professional who knows the person.
Process	Assess for indications that the person thinks he or she can be more self-sufficient. Ask what health professionals have told the person and family. Do their statements seem reasonable? Is the person's description clear and unequivocal? Could the person be more self-sufficient if mood or motivational problems were addressed? Speak with caregivers. What is their perception of the person's capacity? How does this relate to the person's perception and your observations? Assess whether the person's functional performance has recently changed. Has there been an intervening acute episode? What is the likelihood that the person will recover from the current disease or condition?
Coding	0. No
	1. Yes

Example of How to Code Physical Function Improvement Potential

Mrs. S has had Alzheimer's disease resulting in short- and long-term memory loss for several years. She states to the assessor, "I can do everything myself, if they let me." Her daughter states that she must perform all care activities for her mother.

Item G5a should be scored "1" for "Yes".

Item G5b should be scored "0" for "No".

G6.	**Change in ADL Status as Compared to 90 Days Ago, or Since Last Assessment if Less Than 90 Days Ago**
Intent	To determine whether the person's current activities of daily living (ADL) status differs from the status of 90 days ago (or since the last assessment, if that was less than 90 days ago).
Process	Talk to the person. Ask the person to think about how well he or she was able to do ADLs 90 days ago. How does the person's current ADL status compare to 90 days ago? If indicated, talk to a family member or caregiver.
Coding	Code for the most appropriate category. If there is a change in multiple domains, code for the overall direction of change.
	0. Improved
	1. No change
	2. Declined
	3. Uncertain

G7.	**Driving**
Intent	To evaluate one aspect of community independence and determine whether the person's driving is a concern.
Definitions	**G7a. Drove car (vehicle) in the last 90 days** — For example, the person drove to a store, to visit, to a medical appointment.
	G7b. If drove in LAST 90 DAYS, assessor is aware that someone has suggested that person limits OR stops driving.
Process	Ask the person about his or her driving and whether the person plans to continue driving. Be aware that driving may be a sensitive issue. Certain conditions may impair driving ability temporarily or on a more permanent basis. Ask whether the person thinks he or she is able to drive currently. If the person is unsure, recommend that before returning to driving, he or she talk to a physician, take a practice-driving test, or consult an occupational therapist or other appropriate professional(s) to assess driving capacity.
Coding	0. No, or does not drive
	1. Yes

Section H

Continence

H1. Bladder Continence

Intent To determine and record the person's pattern of bladder continence (control) over the last 3 days.

Definition This item describes the person's bladder continence pattern, taking into account any control plans or devices, such as scheduled toileting plans, continence training programs, or urinary appliances. It does not refer to the person's ability to toilet him- or herself—for example, a person may require extensive assistance in toileting and still be continent. Bladder incontinence includes any level of dribbling or wetting of urine.

Process Review the person's urinary elimination pattern with him or her. Make sure that your discussions are held in private. Control of bladder function is a sensitive subject, particularly for persons who are struggling to maintain control. Many persons with poor control will try to hide their problems out of embarrassment or fear of retribution or institutionalization. Others will not report problems because they mistakenly believe that incontinence is a natural part of aging and that nothing can be done to reverse the problem. Despite these common reactions to incontinence, many persons are relieved when a health care professional shows enough concern to ask about the nature of the problem in a sensitive, straightforward manner.

Validate continence patterns with people who know the person well (such as family caregivers).

Remember to consider continence patterns over the last 3-day period, 24 hours a day, including weekends.

Coding A six-level coding scale is used to describe continence patterns. Choose one response to code the person's level of urinary continence over the last 3 days.

0. **Continent** — Complete control, including control achieved by cuing or supervision that involves prompted voiding, habit training, reminders, etc. The person **does not use** any type of catheter or other urinary collection device.

1. **Complete control with any catheter or ostomy** — Control with use of any type of catheter or urinary collection device.

2. **Infrequently incontinent** — Not incontinent over last 3 days, but does have incontinent episodes (i.e., a recent history of incontinence).

3. **Occasionally incontinent** — Less than daily episodes of bladder incontinence (incontinent on 1–2 of the last 3 days).

4. **Frequently incontinent** — Incontinent daily, but some control present (the person is not incontinent during each episode of urination). Example: During the day, the person remains dry and is continent of urine. At night, the person wets his or her bed.

5. **Incontinent** — No control of bladder; multiple daily episodes all or almost all of the time.

8. Did not occur — No urine output from bladder in last 3 days.

Code for the actual bladder continence pattern with urinary device if used. This pattern is the frequency with which the person is wet during the 3-day assessment period. Do not record the level of control that the person **might** have had under optimal circumstances (for example, had a caregiver been available 24 hours/day to help the person with toileting).

If you are uncertain whether to use code **"4"** ("Frequently incontinent") or code **"5"** ("Incontinent"), decide based on the presence (**"4"**) or absence (**"5"**) of any bladder control.

Examples of How to Code Bladder Continence

Mr. Q was taken to the toilet after every meal, before bed, and once during the night. He was never found wet. **Code "0" for "Continent".**

Mr. R had an indwelling catheter in place during the entire 3-day assessment period. He was never found wet. **Code "1" for "Control with any catheter or ostomy".**

Although she is generally continent of urine, every once in a while (4 and 6 days ago over the last week), Mrs. T doesn't make it to the bathroom to urinate in time after receiving her daily diuretic pill. **Code "2" for "Infrequently incontinent".**

Mrs. A has an occasional episode of urinary incontinence (generally less than daily), particularly late in the day when she is tired. In the last 2 days, she was not incontinent at all. She was incontinent 3 days ago, however. **Code "3" for "Occasionally incontinent".**

Mrs. U has end-stage Alzheimer's disease. She is very frail and has stiff, painful contractures of all extremities. She is primarily bedfast on a special water mattress, and is turned and repositioned hourly for comfort. In the last 3 days, she was not toileted and was incontinent of urine for all episodes. **Code "5" for "Incontinent".**

H2. Urinary Collection Device (Excludes Pads/Briefs)

Definitions

External (condom) catheter — A urinary collection device worn over the penis.

Indwelling catheter — A catheter that is maintained within the bladder for the purpose of continuous drainage of urine. Includes catheters inserted through the urethra or by suprapubic incision.

Cystostomy — An opening to the bladder made by a surgical incision and covered by a urinary collection appliance (urostomy bag).

Nephrostomy — A tube, stent, or catheter that is used to provide urinary drainage when a ureter is obstructed. In some cases the catheter drains urine out of a person's body into a drainage bag. In other cases, the catheter drains urine directly into the bladder.

Ureterostomy — A surgical urinary diversion, where the ureter(s) is detached from the bladder and brought to the surface of the abdomen, with a urinary collection device placed over it.

Process

Ask the person or caregiver, and check any clinical documentation. Be sure to ask about any items that are usually hidden from view because they are worn under street clothing (such as a ureterostomy collection bag).

Coding	0. **None**
	1. **Condom catheter**
	2. **Indwelling catheter**
	3. **Cystostomy, nephrostomy, ureterostomy**

H3. Bowel Continence

Intent	To determine and record the person's pattern of bowel continence (control) over the last 3 days.
Definition	The term "bowel continence" refers to control of the person's bowel movements. This item describes the person's bowel continence pattern with any scheduled toileting plans, continence training programs, or appliances in use. It does not refer to the person's ability to toilet him- or herself—for example, a person can require extensive assistance in toileting and still be continent of stool.
Process	The assessment for bowel continence should be completed concurrently with the bladder continence review. Control of bowel function is also a sensitive issue. Be sure to ask about the matter in a sensitive, straightforward manner. If necessary, validate continence patterns with others who know the person (for example, a family member). Remember to consider continence patterns over the **last 3 days, 24 hours a day**.
Coding	0. **Continent** — Complete control; the person **does not use** any type of ostomy device.
	1. **Control with ostomy** — Control with ostomy device over last 3 days.
	2. **Infrequently incontinent** — Not incontinent over last 3 days, but does have incontinent episodes.
	3. **Occasionally incontinent** — Incontinent less than daily.
	4. **Frequently incontinent** — Incontinent daily, but person has some control.
	5. **Incontinent** — No control present.
	8. **Did not occur** — No bowel movement in the last 3 days.

H4. Pads or Briefs Worn

Definition	Any type of absorbent, disposable or reusable undergarment or item, whether worn by the person (for example, a diaper or adult brief) or placed on the bed or chair for protection from incontinence. Does not include the routine use of pads on beds when the person is never or rarely incontinent.
Coding	0. **No**
	1. **Yes**

Section I

Disease Diagnoses

I1. Diseases

Intent

To document the presence of diseases or infections relevant to the person's current ADL status, cognitive status, mood or behavior status, medical treatments, nursing monitoring, or risk of death. In general, these types of conditions are associated with the type and level of care needed by the person. Do not include conditions that have been resolved or no longer affect the person's functioning or care needs.

Definitions

Musculoskeletal

I1a. Hip fracture during last 30 days (or since last assessment if less than 30 days) — Includes any hip fracture that occurred during the past 30 days (or since the last assessment, if that was less than 30 days ago) that continues to have a relationship to current status, treatments, monitoring, etc. Hip fracture diagnoses also include femoral neck fractures, fractures of the trochanter, and subcapital fractures.

I1b. Other fracture over last 30 days (or since last assessment if less than 30 days) — Any fracture other than hip bone (for example, wrist) due to any condition, such as falls or weakening of the bone as a result of cancer.

Neurological

I1c. Alzheimer's disease — A degenerative and progressive dementia that is diagnosed by ruling out other dementias and physiological reasons for the dementia.

I1d. Dementia other than Alzheimer's disease — Includes diagnoses of organic brain syndrome (OBS) or chronic brain syndrome (CBS), senility, senile dementia, multi-infarct dementia, and dementia related to neurological diseases other than Alzheimer's (such as Pick's, Creutzfeldt-Jakob, Huntington's disease, etc.).

I1e. Hemiplegia — Paralysis (temporary or permanent impairment of sensation, function, motion) of both limbs on one side of the body. Usually caused by cerebral hemorrhage, thrombosis, embolism, or tumor. There must be a diagnosis of hemiplegia in the person's record to code this item.

I1f. Multiple sclerosis — A disease in which there is demyelination throughout the central nervous system. Typical symptoms are weakness, uncoordination, paresthesias, speech disturbances, and visual complaints.

I1g. Paraplegia — Paralysis (a temporary or permanent impairment of active motion) of the lower part of the body, including both legs.

I1h. Parkinson's disease — A disorder of the brain characterized by tremor and difficulty with walking, movement, and coordination.

I1i. Quadriplegia — Paralysis (temporary or permanent impairment of sensation, function, motion) of all four limbs and trunk.

I1j. **Stroke/CVA** — A sudden rupture or blockage of a blood vessel within the brain, causing serious bleeding or local obstruction.

Cardiac or Pulmonary

I1k. **Coronary heart disease** — A chronic condition marked by thickening and loss of elasticity of the coronary artery, and caused by deposits of plaque containing cholesterol, lipoid material, and lipophages.

I1l. **Chronic obstructive pulmonary disease** — Any long-standing condition that impairs airflow in and out of the lungs.

I1m. **Congestive heart failure** — A condition in which the heart cannot pump out all the blood that enters it, which leads to an accumulation of blood in the vessels, fluid in the body tissues, and lung congestion.

Psychiatric

I1n. **Anxiety** — A nonpsychotic mental disorder. There are five types, which include:

- Generalized anxiety disorder
- Obsessive-compulsive disorder
- Panic disorder
- Phobias
- Post-traumatic stress disorder

I1o. **Bipolar disorder** — Includes documentation of clinical diagnosis of either manic depression or bipolar disorder. "Bipolar disorder" is the current term for manic-depressive illness.

I1p. **Depression** — A mood disorder often characterized by a depressed mood (for example, the person feels sad or empty, appears tearful); decreased ability to think or concentrate; loss of interest or pleasure in usual activities; insomnia or hypersomnia; loss of energy; change in appetite; or feelings of hopelessness, worthlessness, or guilt. May also include thoughts of death or suicide.

I1q. **Schizophrenia** — A disturbance characterized by delusions, hallucinations, disorganized speech, grossly disorganized behavior, disordered thinking, or flat affect. This category includes schizophrenia subtypes (i.e., paranoid, disorganized, catatonic, undifferentiated, residual).

Infections

I1r. **Pneumonia** — Inflammation of the lungs, most commonly of bacterial or viral origin.

I1s. **Urinary tract infection in last 30 days** — Includes chronic and acute symptomatic infection(s) in the last 30 days. Code only if there is current supporting documentation and significant laboratory findings in the clinical record.

Other

I1t. **Cancer** — Any malignant growth or tumor caused by abnormal and uncontrolled cell division. The malignant growth or tumor may spread to other parts of the body through the lymphatic system or the bloodstream.

I1u. **Diabetes mellitus** — Any of several metabolic disorders marked by persistent thirst and excessive discharge of urine.

Process	Talk to the person and review any available clinical records. Consult with the person's primary physician or nurse practitioner. Talk with family members.
Coding	For all diseases present in Item I1a through Item I1u, select the most appropriate code from those listed below.

0. Not present

1. Primary diagnosis/diagnoses for current stay — One or more diagnoses that are the main reason(s) used to support and justify services being provided.

2. Diagnosis present, receiving active treatment — Treatment can include medications, therapy, or other skilled interventions such as wound care or suctioning.

3. Diagnosis present, monitored but no active treatment — Person has a diagnosis that is being monitored (for example, with laboratory tests or vital signs), but no active treatment is being provided.

I2. Other Disease Diagnoses

Intent	To document the presence of any diseases or infections not listed in Item I1 that are relevant to the person's current ADL status, cognitive status, mood or behavior status, medical treatments, nursing monitoring, or risk of death. Again, do not include conditions that have been resolved or no longer affect the person's functioning or care needs.
Coding	Write the diagnosis on the blank line. Record the appropriate disease code ("**1**", "**2**", or "**3**") in the single box that follows. Then, enter the ICD-CM code in the boxes to the right. You may need to consult a specialist in medical records or medical coding to determine the appropriate ICD-CM code. The ICD code you use may be specific to your country. For example, some countries have begun to use the ICD-10 convention whereas others have not. **NOTE: Add additional lines as necessary for other disease diagnosis.**

Select the most appropriate code from those listed below.

1. Primary diagnosis/diagnoses for current stay — One or more diagnoses that are the main reason(s) used to support and justify services being provided.

2. Diagnosis present, receiving active treatment — Treatment can include medications, therapy, or other skilled interventions such as wound care or suctioning.

3. Diagnosis present, monitored but no active treatment — Person has a diagnosis that is being monitored (for example, with laboratory tests or vital signs), but no active treatment is being provided.

Section J

Health Conditions

J1. Falls

Intent To determine whether the person has a history of falling, which is an important factor in assessing the person's risk of future falls or injuries. Persons who have sustained at least one fall are at risk of future falls. Falls are a common cause of morbidity and mortality among persons receiving home care. Serious injury results from 6% to 10% of falls, with hip fractures accounting for approximately one-half of all serious injuries.

Definition Any unintentional change in position where the person ends up on the floor, ground, or other lower level; includes falls that occur while being assisted by others.

Coding
0. No fall in last 90 days
1. No fall in last 30 days, but fell 31–90 days ago
2. One fall in last 30 days
3. Two or more falls in last 30 days

J2. Recent Falls

NOTE: If the person was last assessed more than 30 days ago, or if this is the person's first assessment, skip this item and proceed to Item J3.

Intent To determine whether the person has a recent history of falling. Asked at follow-up assessment only, and then only if less than 30 days have passed since the last assessment.

Definition **Fall** — Any unintentional change in position where the person ends up on the floor, ground, or other lower level; includes falls that occur while being assisted by others.

Coding If this is the first assessment, or if less than 30 days have passed since the last assessment, simply leave this item blank. If this is a follow-up assessment 30 or more days since the previous assessment, code for the most correct response.

0. No fall in last 30 days
1. Yes, fall in last 30 days

J3. Problem Frequency

Definitions **Balance**

J3a. Difficult or unable to move self to standing position unassisted

J3b. Difficult or unable to turn self around and face the opposite direction when standing

J3c. Dizziness — The person experiences a sensation of unsteadiness, that he or she is turning, or that the surroundings are whirling around.

J3d. Unsteady gait — A gait that places the person at risk of falling. Unsteady gaits take many forms. The person may appear unbalanced or walk with a sway. Other gaits may have uncoordinated or jerking movements. Examples of unsteady gaits include fast gaits with large, careless movements; abnormally slow gaits with small shuffling steps; or wide-based gaits with halting, tentative steps.

Cardiac or Pulmonary

J3e. Chest pain — The person experiences any type of pain in the chest area, which may be described as burning, pressure, stabbing, vague discomfort, etc.

J3f. Difficulty clearing airway secretions — In the last 3 days the person reports being unable, or has been observed to be unable, to cough effectively to expel respiratory secretions (for example, secondary to weakness or pain) or has been unable to mobilize secretions or sputum from mouth (for example, secondary to dysphagia or pain) or tracheostomy (for example, secondary to viscosity of sputum; inability to physically remove secretions from tracheostomy entrance). Examples include a person with pneumonia who is too weak to cough and expel sputum or someone with amyotrophic lateral sclerosis (ALS) who requires suctioning to manage secretions.

Psychiatric

J3g. Abnormal thought process — When the person is observed, there are apparent abnormalities in the form or way in which the person is expressing thoughts. Included are indicators such as loosening of associations, thought blocking, flight of ideas, tangentiality, circumstantiality, clang association, incoherence, neologisms, punning, etc.

> **Loose associations** — The person jumps from one topic to another without an apparent connection between the topics.
>
> **Thought blocking** — The person suddenly stops in the middle of a sentence and is unable to recover what he or she intended to say or to complete other thoughts.
>
> **Flight of ideas** — The person's thoughts are expressed so quickly that the listener has difficulty keeping up.
>
> **Tangentiality** — The person digresses from the subject under discussion and introduces thoughts that seem unrelated, oblique, or irrelevant.
>
> **Circumstantiality** — The person exhibits lack of goal-directedness, incorporates unnecessary details, and has difficulty getting to an end point in the conversation.
>
> **Clang association** — The connection between the person's thoughts is tenuous. The person may use rhyming and punning in his or her speech.
>
> **Incoherence** — The person's speech is unclear or confused. The communication does not make sense to the intended listener.
>
> **Neologism** — The person makes up a word, which may be condensed from several words. Neologisms are unintelligible to the listener.
>
> **Punning** — The person uses words that are similar in sound, but different in meaning.

J3h. **Delusions** — Fixed, false beliefs not shared by others that the person holds even when there is obvious proof or evidence to the contrary. For example, the person may believe that he or she is terminally ill, that his or her spouse is having an affair, or that food served at a restaurant or congregate dining room is poisoned.

J3i. **Hallucinations** — The person has false perceptions that occur in the absence of any real stimuli. A hallucination may be auditory (for example, hearing voices), visual (for example, seeing people or animals), tactile (for example, feeling bugs crawling over the skin), olfactory (for example, smelling poisonous fumes), or gustatory (for example, experiencing strange tastes).

Neurological

J3j. **Aphasia** — A speech or language disorder caused by disease or injury to the brain resulting in difficulty expressing thoughts (speaking or writing) or difficulty understanding spoken or written language.

GI Status

J3k. **Acid Reflux** — The regurgitation of small amounts of acid from the stomach to the throat.

J3l. **Constipation** — No bowel movement in 3 days, or difficult passage of hard stool.

J3m. **Diarrhea** — The frequent elimination of watery stools, regardless of cause.

J3n. **Vomiting** — Regurgitation of stomach contents, regardless of etiology (for example, drug toxicity, influenza, psychogenic).

Sleep Problems

J3o. **Difficulty falling asleep or staying asleep; waking up too early; restlessness; nonrestful sleep** — For example, the person:

- experiences an extended time gap between the point at which he or she attempted to fall asleep and the time at which sleep was actually initiated;
- wakes up well before the desired time due to some factor inherent to him or her (exclude situations in which the person is awakened by some external source);
- experiences sleep that is accompanied by repeated tossing and turning, or dreaming that causes motion or wakefulness, etc., such that the person does not feel relaxed when sleeping and rested when awake; or
- is easily awakened during sleep by sounds or movements, and experiences one or more periods of awakening after sleep is initiated.

J3p. **Too much sleep** — An excessive amount of sleep that interferes with the person's normal functioning.

Other

J3q. **Aspiration** — The inhalation of food or fluid into the person's lungs.

J3r. **Fever** — A rise in the person's body temperature, frequently as a result of infection.

J3s. **GI or GU bleeding** — "Gastrointestinal (GI) bleeding" is any documented bleeding as diagnosed by a gastrointestinal evaluation, or any evidence of current bleeding through rectal exam or guaiac testing. Bleeding may be frank (such as bright red blood) or occult (such as black, guaiac-positive stools). "Genitourinary (GU) bleeding" is bleeding that occurs anywhere along the genitourinary tract. Urine that is dark or cloudy should be tested for the presence of blood. There may also be visible blood in the person's urine or frank, bright red blood coming from the urethral opening.

J3t. **Hygiene** — Unusually poor hygiene, unkempt, disheveled. The person is observed to have unusually poor hygiene well beyond what is considered culturally appropriate. Poor hygiene puts the person at risk for skin breakdown and has other health and psychological ramifications.

J3u. **Peripheral edema** — The person has an abnormal buildup of fluid in foot/ankle/leg tissues.

Process Ask the person—he or she may not have told others of his or her symptoms. Ask family members or caregivers. Review any available clinical records.

Coding
0. Not present
1. Present but not exhibited in last 3 days
2. Exhibited on 1 of last 3 days
3. Exhibited on 2 of last 3 days
4. Exhibited daily in last 3 days

J4. Dyspnea (Shortness of Breath)

Definition The person has reported being, or has been observed to be, breathless or "short of breath."

Process Ask the person if he or she has experienced shortness of breath. If the answer is affirmative, determine if the symptom occurred with strenuous activity, during normal day-to-day activity, or when resting. If the person is unable to respond, review the clinical record and consult with other clinicians and the person's family.

Coding Select the appropriate code from the list below. Code for the most severe occurrence during the last 3 days. If the symptom was absent over the last 3 days, but would have been present had the person undertaken activity, code according to the activity level (day-to-day or moderate) that would normally have caused the person to experience shortness of breath.

"Moderate activities" include some type of physical exercise, such as walking a long distance, climbing 2 flights of stairs, or gardening. "Normal day-to-day activities" include all ADLs (bathing, transferring, etc.) and IADLs (meal preparation, shopping, etc.).

0. Absence of symptom
1. Absent at rest, but present when performed moderate activities
2. Absent at rest, but present when performed normal day-to-day activities
3. Present at rest

J5. Fatigue

Intent
To describe gradations of fatigue or impaired stamina. Fatigue is associated with some chronic diseases and end-stage conditions.

Definitions
Fatigue — An overwhelming or sustained sense of exhaustion resulting in decreased capacity for physical or mental work.

Normal day-to-day activities — These include all ADLs (bathing, transferring, etc.) and IADLs (meal preparation, shopping, etc.).

Coding
Select the appropriate code from the list below. If fatigue was absent over the last 3 days, but would have been present had the person undertaken activity, code according to the activity level that would normally have caused the person to experience fatigue.

0. None

1. Minimal — Diminished energy but completes normal day-to-day activities.

2. Moderate — Due to diminished energy, **unable to finish** normal day-to-day activities.

3. Severe — Due to diminished energy, **unable to start some** normal day-to-day activities.

4. Unable to commence any normal day-to-day activities — Due to diminished energy.

J6. Pain Symptoms

NOTE: Always ask the person about frequency, intensity, and control of the pain. Observe the person and ask others who are in contact with the person.

Intent
To record the frequency and intensity of any pain the person may be experiencing. This item can be used to identify indicators of pain, as well as to monitor the person's response to pain management interventions. A substantial number of persons with pain receive inadequate or no treatment. In particular, persons with chronic, non-cancer-related pain are often overlooked and not treated. One of the biggest reasons for this is that many persons mistakenly believe that pain is to be expected as one ages, or that nothing can be done to relieve their pain.

Definition
Pain — "An unpleasant sensory and emotional experience" that is generally associated with actual or potential tissue damage.

Process
Pain is highly subjective. It is what the person says it is. There are no objective markers or tests to indicate when someone is having pain, or to measure its severity. What a person experiences may not be proportional to the type or extent of the underlying tissue damage. Sometimes a specific cause for chronic pain cannot be identified. Regardless, unless the person refuses, pain must always be treated, even if its cause is unknown.

The most accurate and reliable evidence of the existence of pain and its intensity is what the person tells you. Even in cognitively impaired persons, self-reports of pain should be considered reliable.

However, you may not get an accurate answer if you simply ask "Are you in pain?" A person may think of "pain" as a more intense experience after an acute event—such as what may be experienced after surgery or spraining an ankle. For example, a woman may have a sore foot that "acts up" when she pivots to transfer to her wheelchair or the toilet but that does not bother her most of the time. So she might deny being "in pain". Persons often use different words in describing pain, referring to what they're feeling as "discomfort," " burning," "hurting," "aching," "tightness," "heaviness," "soreness," or a "twinge" or "pang".

If the person states he or she has pain, ask about the degree of control. If the person is unable to tell you if he or she is experiencing some type of painful sensation, observe the person for indicators of pain such as moaning, wincing, or guarding. In some persons, the presence of pain can be hard to discern. For example, persons with dementia may not be able to verbalize that they are feeling pain, although they may manifest pain by particular behaviors such as calling out. Although such behaviors may not be indicative solely of pain, the assessor needs to make a determination (through assessment) if the behaviors are secondary to pain. If necessary, ask those who have had frequent contact with the person whether he or she complained or showed evidence of pain in the last 3 days. However, the person must **first** be asked directly about frequency and intensity.

J6a. **Frequency with which person complains or shows evidence of pain — Including grimacing, teeth clenching, moaning, withdrawal when touched, or other nonverbal signs suggesting pain.**

Coding
0. **No pain**
1. **Present but not exhibited in last 3 days**
2. **Exhibited on 1–2 of last 3 days**
3. **Exhibited daily in last 3 days**

J6b. **Intensity of highest level of pain present — The level of pain reported by or observed in the person.**

Coding
0. **No pain**
1. **Mild**
2. **Moderate**
3. **Severe**
4. **Times when pain is horrible or excruciating**

J6c. **Consistency of pain — Measures the frequency (ebb and flow) of pain from the person's perspective.**

Coding
0. **No pain**
1. **Single episode during last 3 days**
2. **Intermittent**
3. **Constant**

J6d. **Breakthrough pain — The person experienced a sudden, acute flare-up of pain one or more times in the last 3 days. Breakthrough pain might appear as a dramatic increase in the level of** pain above that addressed by ongoing analgesics, or the recurrence of pain associated with end-of-dose failure.

Coding
0. No
1. Yes

J6e. Pain control — The ability of the current therapeutic regimen to control the person's pain adequately (from the person's point of view). This item describes the adequacy or inadequacy of pain control measures (such as medications, massage, TENS, or other therapeutic regimen) instituted by the person, caregiver, or clinical staff caring for the person.

Coding
0. No issue of pain
1. **Pain intensity acceptable to person, no treatment regimen or change in regimen required**
2. **Controlled adequately by therapeutic regimen**
3. **Controlled when therapeutic regimen followed, but not always followed as ordered**
4. **Therapeutic regimen followed, but pain control not adequate**
5. **No therapeutic regimen being followed for pain; pain not adequately controlled**

J7. Instability of Conditions

Definitions

J7a. **Conditions/diseases make cognitive, ADL, mood, or behavior patterns unstable (fluctuating, precarious, or deteriorating)** — For example, the person may have a condition such as ulcerative colitis, rheumatoid arthritis, or multiple sclerosis that causes pain or impairs mobility or sensation, resulting in increased dependence on others and depression.

J7b. **Experiencing an acute episode or a flare-up of a recurrent or chronic problem** — The person is symptomatic for an acute health condition (such as new myocardial infarction, adverse drug reaction, or influenza) or recurrent acute condition (such as aspiration pneumonia or urinary tract infection). Also included are persons who are experiencing an exacerbation or flare-up of a chronic condition (for example, new-onset shortness of breath in someone with a history of asthma, or increased pedal edema in a person with congestive heart failure). This type of acute episode usually is of sudden onset, has a time-limited course, and requires evaluation by a physician.

J7c. **End-stage disease, 6 or fewer months to live** — The person or family has been told that in the best clinical judgment of the physician, the person has end-stage disease with approximately 6 or fewer months to live.

Process
Consult with the person and the person's family. Review any clinical records. Use your clinical judgment to determine whether it is appropriate to ask the person about whether they have an "end-stage disease" (Item J7c).

Coding
0. No
1. Yes

J8. Self-Reported Health

Process Ask the person: "In general, how would you rate your health?" Record the person's response according to one of the categories below. Do not code based on your own inferences about the person's physical health and do not record ratings given by family, friends, or other informants. This item should be treated strictly as a self-report measure. If the person is unable (for example, due to cognitive impairment) or refuses to respond, do not dwell on the item and do not presume responses for the person; instead, code that the person could not/would not respond.

Coding
0. **Excellent**
1. **Good**
2. **Fair**
3. **Poor**
8. **Could not (would not) respond**

J9. Tobacco and Alcohol

J9a. Smokes tobacco daily

Intent To determine whether the person smokes tobacco.

Definition **Tobacco** — Refers to cigar, cigarette, or any other tobacco product that is inhaled.

Process Ask the person directly. This information may be sensitive to the person or create feelings within the assessor. Care must be taken to acknowledge these feelings. Begin asking the person about tobacco usage, with a simple nonjudgmental question, "Do you smoke?" If yes, determine the frequency. Address this issue in a gentle way to avoid the person feeling judged or that he or she is doing something wrong. For example, you might say "Like the other questions I asked, I am just trying to find out about you . . . it doesn't mean that what you are doing is wrong." Validate tobacco usage with a family member or caregiver. This discussion should not take place in front of the person.

Coding
0. **No**
1. **Not in last 3 days, but is usually a daily smoker**
2. **Yes**

J9b. Alcohol

Intent To determine if a person's consumption of alcohol is a potential problem by identifying the highest number of alcoholic drinks the person had in a "single sitting" during **the last 14 days.**

Definitions **Alcohol** — Includes beer, wine, mixed drinks, liquor, and liqueurs.

Single sitting — Refers to any given point in time (for example, at dinner, after work, while out at a social event, watching television).

Process Ask the person directly about whether he or she consumes alcohol. Consult with a family member if necessary. Sometimes it is prudent to talk to the person and family separately. Start by asking the person, "Do you drink alcoholic drinks?" If he or she says yes, then ask, "When you look back over the last 14 days, what is the highest number of drinks you had in a single sitting?"

Coding Code for the highest number of drinks ingested by the person at one sitting over the last 14 days.

   0. None

   1. 1

   2. 2–4

   3. 5 or more

Section K

Oral and Nutritional Status

K1. **Height and Weight [Country Specific]**

NOTE: If not in the USA, please consult your addendum regarding measurements.

Intent
To record the person's current height and weight in order to monitor nutrition, hydration status, and weight stability over time. For example, a person who has had edema may experience an expected weight loss as a result of taking a diuretic. Weight loss can also be the intended result of limiting caloric intake and participating in an exercise program, or the unintended consequence of poor intake and malnutrition.

Record **height in inches** (Item K1a) and **weight in pounds** (Item K1b). Base weight on most recent measure in the last 30 days.

K1a. **Height**

Process
Measure height in inches with a tape measure or other device. If the last recorded height was more than 1 year ago, measure the person's height again. Wherever possible, use a calibrated measure. In its absence, use estimates from the person, family member, or caregiver.

Round height up to nearest whole inch. Measure height consistently over time in accordance with standard agency practice (shoes off, etc.).

Coding
Enter one digit in each box.

K1b. **Weight**

Process
Base weight on most recent weight measured within the last 30 days. Round the person's weight upward to the nearest whole pound. Measure weight consistently over time in accordance with standard agency practice (after voiding, before meal, etc.). Wherever possible use a calibrated scale. In its absence, use estimates from the person, family member, or caregiver.

Coding
Enter one digit in each box. If the person weighs less than 100 pounds, use "0" as a filler digit in the first box.

K2. **Nutritional Issues**

Intent
Marked, unintended declines in weight can indicate failure to thrive; a sign of a potentially serious medical problem; or poor nutritional intake due to physical, cognitive, or social factors.

K2a.	**Weight loss of 5% or more in LAST 30 DAYS, or 10% or more in LAST 180 DAYS**
Process	Ask the person or family about weight changes over the last 30 and 180 days. Use actual records of weight if available. A subjective estimate of weight change from the person or caretaker can be used if no written records are available. Identifying a particular time approximately 6 months earlier (such as "compared to last New Year's") may help the person remember his or her approximate weight 180 days ago. You may be able to help the person answer the question by asking "How much weight do you think you have lost?"; then mentally compare this with the reported or your estimated current weight of the person. You can also ask, "Have you lost a lot of weight? Do you feel much thinner or weaker?" or "Your clothes seem very loose on you. Were you much heavier 6 months ago?"
K2b.	**Dehydrated or BUN/creatinine ratio > 25 (this ratio is country specific)**
Process	Identifying dehydration can be difficult. Record your clinical judgment based upon signs and symptoms (for example, severe vomiting over a period of time). Alternatively, laboratory results indicating dehydration may be available (i.e., BUN/creatinine ratio of >25 [note that the standard for this ratio value can be country specific]).
K2c.	**Fluid intake less than four 8 oz cups per day (or less than 1,000 cc per day)**
Definition	Person did not consume all/almost all fluids during the last 3 days.
K2d.	**Fluid output exceeds input**
Definition	Fluid loss exceeds the amount of fluids the person takes in (for example, loss from vomiting, fever, or diarrhea that exceeds fluid replacement).
K3.	**Mode of Nutritional Intake**
Intent	The ability to swallow safely can be affected by many disease processes and by functional decline. Alterations in one's ability to swallow could result in choking and aspiration, both of which can cause morbidity and mortality. Often persons with swallowing difficulties require altered consistencies of food and fluids in order to ingest nutrition by mouth. This item details any dietary modifications necessary to address swallowing difficulties.
Process	Observe and talk with the person. If available, review the person's clinical record, including MD, dietitian, and speech-language pathology notes if applicable.
Coding	Using the codes provided, indicate which item best describes the dietary prescription used to accommodate swallowing difficulties. **0. Normal** — Person swallows all types of foods. **1. Modified independent** — For example, liquid is sipped, or person takes limited solid food; need for modification may be unknown.

2. **Requires diet modification to swallow solid food** — For example, mechanical diet (puree, minced, etc.) is required, or person is only able to ingest specific foods.

3. **Requires modification to swallow liquids** — For example, liquids must be thickened.

4. **Can swallow only pureed solids AND thickened liquids**

5. **Combined oral and parenteral or tube feeding**

6. **Nasogastric tube feeding only**

7. **Abdominal feeding tube** — For example, a PEG tube.

8. **Parenteral feeding only** — Includes all types of parenteral feedings, such as total parenteral nutrition (TPN).

9. **Activity did not occur** — Person did not eat or receive any form of nutritional supplementation during the last 3 days.

K4. Dental or Oral

Intent To record any oral problems present in the last 3 days.

Definitions

K4a. **Wears a denture (removable prosthesis)** — The person wears a device that may replace all or some of the teeth of the upper or lower jaw. A denture is removable by the person or a helper.

K4b. **Has broken, fragmented, loose, or otherwise nonintact natural teeth** — The person has natural teeth that are broken, fragmented (i.e., a piece of tooth is missing), or loose (i.e., tooth is movable when touched).

K4c. **Reports having dry mouth** — The person reports having a dry mouth or difficulty in moving a food bolus in his or her mouth.

K4d. **Reports difficulty chewing** — The person is unable to chew food easily and without pain or difficulties, regardless of cause (for example, the person might use ill-fitting dentures, or have a neurologically impaired chewing mechanism, temporomandibular joint pain, or a painful tooth).

Process Ask the person about difficulties in these areas. If possible, observe the person during a meal. Inspect the mouth for abnormalities that could contribute to chewing or swallowing problems or mouth pain.

Coding

0. No
1. Yes

Section L

Skin Condition

Intent — To determine the condition of the person's skin, identify the presence and stage of ulcers, document other skin conditions, and note any foot problems that may be present.

L1. **Most Severe Pressure Ulcer**

Intent — To record the highest stage of pressure ulcers on any part of the body present in the last 3 days.

Definition — **Pressure ulcer** — Any lesion caused by unrelieved pressure. Pressure ulcers usually occur over bony prominences and are staged to classify the degree of tissue damage observed.

Process — Consult with the person and family about the presence of an ulcer. If an ulcer exists, the assessor may have to observe the ulcer to determine its stage (see "Coding" below).

Ask if the person has been examined for the presence of pressure ulcers or other skin conditions. It could be difficult to examine the person's entire skin, as you are a guest in the person's home. For persons who are cognitively intact, you can get good information about their skin condition without conducting a skin examination. For a chair-bound or bedfast person, conduct a skin examination, paying particular attention to the person's hips, thighs, buttocks, low back, and heels.

It is sometimes difficult to determine the presence of a reddened area (a Stage 1 ulcer) in persons with darker skin tones. To recognize Stage 1 ulcers, look for:

- Any change in the feel of the tissue in a high-risk area;
- Any change in the appearance of the skin in high-risk areas, such as an "orange-peel" look or a subtle purplish hue; and
- Extremely dry crust-like areas that, upon closer examination, are found to cover a tissue break.

Coding

0. **No pressure ulcer**

1. **Any area of persistent skin redness** — An area of skin that appears continually reddened and does not disappear when pressure is relieved. There is no break in the skin. Also known as "Stage 1."

2. **Partial loss of skin layers** — A partial-thickness loss of skin that presents clinically as an abrasion, blister, or shallow crater. Also known as "Stage 2."

3. **Deep craters in the skin** — A full thickness of skin is lost, exposing the subcutaneous tissues. Presents as a deep crater with or without undermining of adjacent tissue. Also known as "Stage 3."

4. **Breaks in skin exposing muscle or bone** — A full thickness of skin and subcutaneous tissue is lost, exposing muscle or bone. Also known as "Stage 4."

5. **Not codable** — For example, because necrotic eschar is predominant.

L2. Prior Pressure Ulcer

Intent
To document a history of pressure ulcers, which is a risk factor for the development of pressure ulcers in the future.

Process
Ask the person if he or she has ever had a pressure ulcer that is now healed. A review of old records (including discharge summaries), clinical progress notes, flow sheets, or care plans may also yield this information. If necessary, check with a family member or care provider who has prior knowledge of the person's skin condition.

Coding
Select the appropriate response.

0. No
1. Yes

L3. Presence of Skin Ulcer Other Than Pressure Ulcer

Intent
To identify the presence of any skin ulcer that is not a pressure ulcer—for example, a venous ulcer, arterial ulcer, mixed venous-arterial ulcer, or diabetic foot ulcer.

Definition
An open lesion caused by poor circulation in the lower limbs.

Coding
Select the appropriate response.

0. No
1. Yes

L4. Major Skin Problems

Definitions
Major skin problems — This item includes lesions, second- or third-degree burns, and healing surgical wounds.

Burn — Injury to tissues resulting from thermal, electrical, chemical, or radioactive exposure. The effect of the injury may be local or systemic.

Coding
Code for the appropriate response.

0. No
1. Yes

L5. Skin Tears or Cuts (Other Than Surgery)

Definition
Any traumatic break in the skin penetrating to the subcutaneous tissue. Does not include surgical incisions.

Coding
Code for the appropriate response.

0. No
1. Yes

L6. Other Skin Conditions or Changes in Skin Condition

Intent
To document the presence of skin problems other than ulcers, skin tears, or cuts and the major skin problems represented in the earlier items.

Definitions
Other skin conditions or changes in skin condition — For example, bruises, rashes, itching, mottling, herpes zoster, intertrigo, or eczema.

Rash — A transient eruption of the skin.

Mottling — A condition characterized by areas of skin discoloration.

Eczema — Major features include pruritus, atypical morphology and distribution, and a tendency toward dry skin and itching. Flaking of skin may occur.

Coding
Code for the appropriate response.

0. No
1. Yes

L7. Foot Problems

Definition
Includes bunions, hammertoes, overlapping toes, structural problems, infections, and ulcers.

Coding
Code for the appropriate response.

0. **No foot problems**
1. **Foot problems, no limitation in walking**
2. **Foot problems limit walking**
3. **Foot problems prevent walking**
4. **Foot problems, does not walk for other reasons**

Section M

Medications

M1. List of All Medications

Intent To facilitate a medication evaluation by having a single listing of all prescribed and nonprescribed medications taken by the person. This section will help clinicians identify potential problems related to the consumption of, or failure to take, medications (such as any physical or emotional problems an individual may experience as the result of taking one or more medications). For example, identifying how frequently an individual uses a PRN (as needed) pain medication, sleeping medication, or laxative may lead the clinician to do further assessment of underlying problems that prompted their use. It may also help the clinician identify medications that might cause specific problems such as incontinence or delirium.

Definitions **Medications** — These include all prescribed, nonprescribed, and over-the-counter medications that the person consumed in the last 3 days. Medications may be taken by mouth, placed on the skin or in the eyes, injected, given intravenously, etc. This includes prescriptions now discontinued but taken in the last 3 days and drugs prescribed PRN (as needed) that were taken during this period. It also includes medications that are prescribed on a maintenance schedule, such as vitamin injections given once a month, even if they were not given in the last 3 days.

Drug code — These codes may vary depending on what country you are in. For example, some but not all countries use the National Drug Code (NDC), which is a standardized system for coding medications. An individual NDC code provides information on the drug name, dose, and form of the drug.

For additional definitions of terms under Item M1, see the individual explanations for M1a through M1g.

Process Ask the person, and family members when appropriate, to list all medications actually taken in the last 3 days. Be certain to specify that this is not just prescription medication, but any medication consumed, regardless of how it was obtained.

Ask the person or family member to get out all the medications the person is currently using or has used in the last 3 days. It will help to have the actual drug container, so you can get the proper spelling of the drug name and accurate dosage and frequency. If the person cannot actually get the medications out on his or her own, offer to retrieve them. While you are documenting the medications for the assessment, review the schedule of medications with the person to verify when and how often he or she takes each medication. However, be sure to tell the person that you need to know about all medications he or she has taken (prescription and others), regardless of how they were obtained. In some cases, it may be possible to get a printout from the person's pharmacy of all current drug prescriptions. If so, confirm that the list is current; that the person is actually taking each prescription, especially those listed as PRN (as needed); and that the person gets his or her drugs only from this pharmacy. In addition, ask the person if he or she (or someone on his/her behalf) visited the drugstore to get any over-the-counter medications. Ask if the person is taking any specific drugs for problem conditions he or she may have mentioned to you (such as constipation, allergies, skin rashes, or fungus infections). The person may also have visited a doctor in the past few days, in which case you can ask whether any medications were changed. If so, determine which ones were added or discontinued. Do not record new medications unless the person has already begun taking them during the assessment period.

Record all medications that the person **received** (actually swallowed, inhaled, injected, or applied to skin, eyes, etc.) in the last 3 days. Also record any prescribed medications that may not have been consumed in the last 3 days, but are part of the person's regular medication regimen (such as monthly B_{12} injections).

Count only those PRN (as needed) medications that were actually taken by the person in the last 3 days.

In recording the information on the form or in the computer, be sure to check the list of medications twice, so that you do not miss any. Make sure you count medications that may have been discontinued, but were administered in the last 3 days.

NOTE: Herbal preparations in all forms (pills, liquids, powders, teas, etc.) should not be included in Item M1, "List of All Medications". According to the U.S. Food and Drug Administration, herbal preparations are considered nutritional supplements and not medications.

The coding instructions for Item M1 are extensive. Review them carefully, from M1a through M1g; for each drug record, you will need to enter information in all the columns (M1a, M1b, and so forth). Complete the coding exercise at the end of all the explanations of this item.

M1a. Name

Definition

The name of the medication. Either the generic name or the trade name is acceptable.

Coding

In the first column of the table on the Assessment Form, write the name of the medication exactly as it appears on the medication container. For an illustration of how this should be coded, see "Example of How to Code Medication Name, Dose, and Unit" under M1c.

M1b. Dose

Definition

The dose received. This is a positive number—for example, 0.5, 5, 150, or 300.

Coding

In the column under "Dose", record the dose that was ordered by the physician **exactly** as it appears on the medication container. For example, if the medication label indicates "Acetaminophen 650 mg", do not write "Acetaminophen 325 mg 2 tabs"—even if two 325 mg tablets were actually taken by the person. **NOTE: Never write a zero by itself after a decimal point—"X mg" is correct (not "X.0 mg"). Always use a zero before a decimal point—"0.X mg" is correct (not ".X mg").**

Occasionally, dosages of medication may have changed during the 3-day assessment period. In this case, each dosage of the medication should be recorded separately.

For an illustration of how this should be coded, see "Example of How to Code Medication Name, Dose, and Unit" under M1c.

M1c. **Unit**

Coding Use the following list to record the unit.

gtts	(drops)	**mEq**	(milliequivalent)	**puffs**	
gm	(gram)	**mg**	(milligram)	**%**	(percent)
L	(liter)	**mL**	(milliliter)	**units**	
mcg	(microgram)	**oz**	(ounce)	**oth**	(other)

Example of How to Code Medication Name, Dose, and Unit

List obtained by reviewing a person's medication containers and verifying they were taken during the assessment period of August 11, 2005–August 13, 2005

- Lasix 40 mg daily po
- Acetaminophen 325 mg 2 tabs q3–4 hrs PRN by mouth (given 3 times in last 3 days)
- B$_{12}$ 1 cc every month by injection (given August 8, 2005)
- Isopto Carbachol 1.5% 2 drops left eye tid (3 times a day)
- Robitussin DM 5 cc at bedtime as needed po (not given last 3 days)
- Motrin 400 mg qid by mouth (given August 11, 2005)
- Dilantin 300 mg at bedtime, by mouth (given August 11, 2005)

a. Name	b. Dose	c. Unit	d. Route	e. Freq.	f. PRN	g. ATC or NDC code
Lasix	40	mg				
Acetaminophen	650	mg				
B$_{12}$	1	mL				
Isopto Carbachol 1.5%	2	gtts				
Motrin	400	mg				
Dilantin	300	mg				

Note that Robitussin DM was not recorded because it was not taken in last 3 days.

M1d. **Route of administration**

Coding Use the following list to record the route of administration.

po	(by mouth/oral)	**sub-q**	(subcutaneous)	**nas**	(nasal)
sl	(sublingual)	**rec**	(rectal)	**et**	(enteral tube)
im	(intramuscular)	**top**	(topical)	**td**	(transdermal)
iv	(intravenous)	**ih**	(inhalation)	**oth**	(other)

Example for Route of Administration

Medication list obtained from medication review with the person (for assessment period August 11, 2005–August 13, 2005)

- Mylanta 15 cc after meals, by mouth
- Zantac one tab (150 mg) every 12 hours via G-tube
- Transderm nitro patch 2.5, 1 patch daily (apply to skin)
- Humulin N 15 units before breakfast daily sq
- Lasix 80 mg intravenous
- Acetaminophen suppository, one via the rectum (650 mg) every 4 hours as needed (given on two occasions in last 3 days)

a. Name	b. Dose	c. Unit	d. Route	e. Freq.	f. PRN	g. ATC or NDC code
Mylanta	15	cc	**po**			
Zantac	150	mg	**et**			
Transderm nitro patch 2.5	1	oth	**td**			
Humulin N	15	units	**sub-q**			
Lasix	80	mg	**iv**			
Acetaminophen supp.	650	mg	**rec**			

M1e. **Frequency**

Definition The number of times per day, week, or month the medication is taken.

Coding Use the list that follows. For an illustration of how this should be coded, see "Example of How to Code Frequency and PRN" under M1f.

q1h	(every hour)	**q2d**	(every other day)
q2h	(every 2 hours)	**q3d**	(every 3 days)
q3h	(every 3 hours)	**weekly**	
q4h	(every 4 hours)	**2w**	(2 times weekly)
q6h	(every 6 hours)	**3w**	(3 times weekly)
q8h	(every 8 hours)	**4w**	(4 times weekly)
daily		**5w**	(5 times weekly)
bed	(at bedtime)	**6w**	(6 times weekly)
bid	(2 times daily; includes every 12 hours)	**1m**	(monthly)
tid	(3 times daily)	**2m**	(twice every month)
qid	(4 times daily)	**oth**	(other)
5d	(5 times daily)		

M1f. **PRN**

Definition Medication given as needed or "SOS".

Coding 0. No
1. Yes

Example of How to Code Frequency and PRN

Medication list obtained by reviewing all the person's medications with him or her (for assessment period of August 14, 2005–August 16, 2005)

- Ampicillin 250 mg every 6 hours for 10 days, by mouth (starting on August 10)
- Beconase nasal inhaler 1 puff twice a day
- Compazine suppository 5 mg as needed for nausea (taken on August 15)
- Lanoxin 0.25 mg every other day, by mouth. On alternate days, take Lanoxin 0.125 mg
- Peri-Colace two capsules at bedtime, by mouth
- Humulin N 15 units before breakfast daily sq. Check blood sugar daily at 4 p.m. Sliding-scale insulin: Humulin R 5 units if blood sugar 200–300; 10 units if over 300. (5 units given on August 14 for blood sugar of 255; 10 units given on August 16 for blood sugar of 305)
- (Over-the-counter) Claritin one tablet (10 mg) each day, taken three times in the last 3 days

a. Name	b. Dose	c. Unit	d. Route	e. Freq.	f. PRN	g. ATC or NDC code
Ampicillin	250	mg	po	q6h	0	
Beconase	1	puffs	nas	bid	0	
Compazine suppository	5	mg	rec	q3d	1	
Lanoxin	0.25	mg	po	q2d	0	
Lanoxin	0.125	mg	po	q2d	0	
Peri-Colace	0.125	mg	po	bed	0	
Humulin N	15	units	sub-q	daily	0	
Humulin R	5	units	sub-q	q3d	0	
Humulin R	10	units	sub-q	q3d	0	
Claritin	10	mg	po	daily	0	

M1g.

Coding

National Drug Code (ATC or NDC code)

It is important that all of the information about the medication (medication name, dose ordered, frequency, and amount administered) correspond with the NDC code. A medication usually has more than one NDC code. The different types of NDC codes are based on the **strength** of the medication and the **form** of the medication (solution, tablets, ampules, syringes, ointment, cream, vial, spray, drops, etc.). For example, there are twenty-one NDC codes for morphine. If a person were receiving 2 mg of morphine im and the pharmacy sent it in an ampule form, the NDC code would be 006411180; if the pharmacy sent the morphine in a vial, the NDC code would be 006412343. If you obtain a printout from the pharmacist, you may be able to obtain the NDC code from that printout.

There will be occasions when a medication dosage will involve two NDC codes. For example, if Coumadin 3 mg were ordered, the pharmacy would send a 1 mg tablet and a 2 mg tablet, each having a different NDC code. In cases such as this, use the NDC code for the largest dose (2 mg).

Code investigational drugs as 999999999. Code compounds (topical mixtures prepared by the pharmacist) as 888888888.

Record the NDC code in column g. There should be nine (9) digits in the NDC code. Recheck the number to be sure you have entered the digits correctly. Many NDC codes begin with one or more zeros. These zeros are important; do not omit them. If the NDC codes you are using have eleven (11) digits, disregard the last two digits, as these are the package codes.

Example of How to Score NDC Codes

Medication list obtained from review of all medications with the person (for assessment period of August 11, 2005–August 13, 2005)

- Lanoxin one tablet (0.125 mg) daily, by mouth
- Haldol 1 mg liquid every 8 hrs as needed, by mouth (administered two times in last 3 days)
- Ampicillin liquid 250 mg every 6 hrs by mouth
- Acetaminophen 650 mg four times a day, by mouth (pharmacy supplies two 325 mg tablets)
- Humulin N 15 units before breakfast daily sq
- Check blood sugar daily at 4 p.m. Sliding-scale insulin: Humulin R 5 units if blood sugar 200–300; 10 units if over 300. (5 units given on August 11 for BS of 255; 5 units given on August 13 for BS of 233)
- Transderm nitro 1 patch once a day, apply to the skin
- Diazepam 3 mg at bedtime, by mouth

a. Name	b. Dose	c. Unit	d. Route	e. Freq.	f. PRN	g. ATC or NDC code
Lanoxin	0.125	mg	po	daily	0	0 0 0 8 1 0 2 4 2
Haldol	1	mg	po	q2d	1	0 0 0 5 6 0 2 5 0
Ampicillin	250	mg	po	q6h	0	0 0 0 4 7 2 3 0 2
Acetaminophen	650	mg	po	qid	0	0 0 7 8 1 1 2 9 4
Humulin N	15	units	sub-q	daily	0	0 0 0 0 2 8 3 1 5
Humulin R	5	units	sub-q	q2d	0	0 0 0 0 2 8 2 1 5
Transderm nitro	1	oth	td	daily	0	0 0 0 8 3 2 0 2 5
Diazepam	3	mg	po	bed	0	0 0 3 6 4 0 7 7 4

Coding Exercise for Item M1

This exercise is designed to give you practice in completing Item M1 all the way through, from M1a to M1g. Using the list of medications below, fill in the blank table on the next page. When you have finished, compare your entries to the table on the following page, which is already filled in and coded correctly.

The 3-day assessment period for the exercise is September 1, 2005–September 3, 2005.

- Inderal 40 mg twice a day, by mouth
- Artificial tears 1 drop to each eye, four times a day
- Anusol-HC suppository 1 via rectum as needed (given one time in last 3 days)
- Amoxicillin 500 mg every 6 hours through the G-tube
- Benylin cough syrup 2 tablespoons every 4 hours as needed by mouth (given ten times in last 3 days)
- Darvocet-N 100 2 tabs every 4–6 hrs as needed, by mouth (given a total of five times in last 3 days)
- Heparin lock flush 10 units daily
- Ditropan syrup 2.5 mg daily, by mouth
- Nitro Transdermal 0.4 mg 1 patch (apply to skin) daily
- Novolin N 24 units before breakfast sq
- Check blood sugar before breakfast. Sliding-scale insulin: Novolin R 10 units if blood sugar over 200 (10 units given on 2 days in last 3 days)
- Questran 1 packet with each meal by mouth
- Quinine sulfate 325 mg one capsule at bedtime
- Coumadin 2.5 mg one tablet daily, by mouth (discontinued September 3, 2005)
- Coumadin 5 mg one tablet daily, by mouth (ordered to start on September 4, 2005)
- Maalox 15 cc as needed for indigestion by mouth (not administered in last 3 days)

a. Name	b. Dose	c. Unit	d. Route	e. Freq.	f. PRN	g. ATC or NDC code

Compare your responses with the correctly scored table on the next page.

a. Name	b. Dose	c. Unit	d. Route	e. Freq.	f. PRN	g. ATC or NDC code
Inderal	40	mg	po	bid	0	0 0 0 4 6 0 4 2 4
Artificial tears	1	gtts	top	qid	0	0 0 3 4 9 8 6 1 5
Anusol-HC suppository	1	oth	rec	oth	1	0 0 0 7 1 1 0 8 8
Amoxicillin	500	mg	et	q6h	0	0 0 3 0 4 0 5 8 7
Benylin cough syrup	2	units	po	tid	1	0 0 0 7 1 2 1 9 5
Darvocet-N 100	200	mg	po	bid	1	0 0 0 0 2 0 3 6 3
Heparin lock flush	10	units	iv	daily	0	0 0 4 6 9 3 0 0 1
Ditropan syrup	2.5	mg	po	daily	0	0 0 0 8 8 1 3 7 3
Nitro Transdermal	0.4	mg	td	daily	0	4 7 2 0 2 2 8 3 2
Novolin N	24	units	sub-q	daily	0	0 0 0 0 3 1 8 3 4
Novolin R	10	units	sub-q	q2d	0	0 0 0 0 3 1 8 3 3
Questran	1	oth	po	tid	0	0 0 0 8 7 0 5 8 0
Quinine sulfate	325	mg	po	bed	0	0 0 0 0 2 0 6 2 9
Coumadin	2.5	mg	po	daily	0	0 0 0 5 6 0 1 7 6

Note that Maalox was not recorded because it was not taken during the assessment period in the last 3 days. Similarly, the 5 mg dosage of Coumadin was not recorded because it was not taken during the assessment period—it was not scheduled to be taken until the following day.

M2.	**Allergy to Any Drug**
Intent	To determine if the individual has any known allergies to either prescription or over-the-counter medications.
Definition	The presence of an allergy would be determined by a history of a serious negative reaction to a particular drug or category of drugs.
Process	Ask the person whether he or she is allergic or has ever had a reaction to any drug(s). Include reactions to both prescription and over-the-counter drugs administered by any route.
Coding	Select the appropriate code. **0. No known drug allergies** **1. Yes**

M3.	**Adherent with Medications Prescribed by Physician**
Intent	To determine if the person is receiving medications as prescribed by a physician, nurse practitioner, or physician's assistant.
Definition	The person is actually taking medications **as prescribed**.
Process	You will have already solicited information from the person about his or her medications. Compare the person's responses with available medication and known medication orders. Does the supply remaining seem appropriate considering when the prescription was filled? Did the person and caregiver give accurate information about medication administration? Remember, this item is not intended to evaluate the appropriateness of the medication prescribed.
Coding	**0. Always adherent** **1. Adherent 80% of time or more** — Over the last 3 days, 24 hours a day, the person deviated from prescribed medication regime 20% or less of the time. **2. Adherent less than 80% of the time, including failure to purchase prescribed medications** — Over the last 3 days, 24 hours a day, person deviated from prescribed medication regime more than 20% of the time. **8. No medications prescribed** — Person is not receiving any prescribed medication.

Section N

Treatments and Procedures

N1. Prevention

Intent This item helps home care workers to identify whether the person has unmet needs for health counseling and preventive care.

Process Ask the person if he or she received the following specific health measures.

N1a. Blood pressure measured in LAST YEAR — The person's blood pressure was measured by a clinician during the past year.

N1b. Colonoscopy test in LAST 5 YEARS — The entire colon (from anus to cecum) was viewed by means of a fiber-optic colonoscope.

N1c. Dental exam in LAST YEAR — The person underwent a dental examination by a dentist, oral surgeon, or dental hygienist during the past year.

N1d. Eye exam in LAST YEAR — The person underwent an eye examination by an ophthalmologist, optometrist, physician, nurse, or other clinician within the past year.

N1e. Hearing exam in LAST 2 YEARS — The person underwent a hearing examination by an audiologist or other clinician within the past 2 years.

N1f. Influenza vaccine in LAST YEAR — The person has received vaccination for influenza prevention during the past year.

N1g. Mammogram or breast exam in LAST 2 YEARS (for women) — The person had either a mammogram or a breast examination by a clinician during the past 2 years.

N1h. Pneumovax vaccine in LAST 5 YEARS or after age 65 — The person received the vaccine for prevention of pneumonia within the past 5 years or after age 65.

Coding Code the appropriate response.

0. No
1. Yes

N2. Treatments and Programs Received or Scheduled in the Last 3 Days (or Since Last Assessment if Less Than 3 Days)

Intent To review prescribed treatments and determine the extent of the person's adherence to the prescription. This item includes special treatments, therapies, and programs received or scheduled during the last 3 days (or since the last assessment if less than 3 days have passed), as well as adherence to the required schedule. It includes services received in the home or on an outpatient basis.

Definitions

Treatments

N2a. Chemotherapy — Includes any type of chemotherapy (anticancer drug) given by any route.

N2b. Dialysis — Includes peritoneal or renal dialysis that occurs at home or at a facility.

N2c. Infection control — For example, isolation or quarantine. Enforced isolation or restriction of free movement imposed to prevent the spread of a contagious disease.

N2d. IV medication — Includes any drug or biological (for example, contrast material) given by intravenous push or drip through a central or peripheral port. Does not include a saline or heparin flush to keep a heparin lock patent, or IV fluids without medication.

N2e. Oxygen therapy — Includes continuous or intermittent oxygen via mask, cannula, etc.

N2f. Radiation — Includes radiation therapy or having a radiation implant.

N2g. Suctioning — Includes oropharyngeal, nasopharyngeal, or tracheal aspiration.

N2h. Tracheostomy care — Includes removal of cannula and cleansing of tracheostomy site and surrounding skin with appropriate solutions.

N2i. Transfusion — Includes transfusion of whole blood or any type of blood products.

N2j. Ventilator or respirator — Mechanical device designed to provide adequate ventilation in persons who are, or may become, unable to support their own respiration. Includes any type of electrically or pneumatically powered closed-system mechanical ventilatory support devices. Includes any person who was in the process of being weaned off the ventilator or respirator in the last 3 days.

N2k. Wound care — Includes the application of bandages (for example, dry gauze dressings, dressings moistened with saline or other solutions, transparent dressings, hydrogel dressings, or dressings with hydrocolloid or hydroactive particles); wound irrigation; the application of ointments and topical medications to treat skin conditions (for example, cortisone, antifungal preparations, or chemotherapeutic agents); debridement (chemical or surgical) to remove dirt or dead tissue from a wound; and suture removal.

Programs

N2l. Scheduled toileting program — The person is taken to the toilet room, given a urinal, or reminded to go to the toilet on a regular and ongoing basis. In the home, this may be done by family members or paid help. Includes any habit training or prompted voiding program.

N2m. Palliative care program — A formal program in which care is focused on the relief of pain and other uncomfortable symptoms (such as dyspnea). Persons receiving palliative care generally have end-stage disease, but may or may not have a prognosis of 6 months or less to live (i.e., the person may live for many months or years).

N2n. Turning/repositioning program — The person is periodically turned from side to side and onto his or her back while in bed. Once the person has been turned to the new side, staff ensures that the head, torso, and limbs are positioned to minimize pain, promote function, and minimize pressure on bony prominences.

Process	Ask the person if he or she received specific treatments or programs.
Coding	0. **Not ordered AND did not occur**
	1. **Ordered, not implemented**
	2. **1–2 of last 3 days**
	3. **Daily in last 3 days**

N3. Formal Care — Days and Total Minutes of Care in Last 7 Days

Intent	To capture the number of minutes spent by formal caregiving agencies in providing care or care management in the last 7 days (or since the last assessment or admission, if less than 7 days have passed).
Definitions	**Care** — Includes direct services provided to the person (both ADL and IADL support), the management of care received (for example, making medication schedules, planning for future needs), and the provision of therapeutic care by any formal agency or service provider.

- **N3a.** **Home health aide** — Aides who traditionally provide "hands-on" ADL support and simple monitoring (such as taking blood pressure).
- **N3b.** **Home nurse** — Licensed or registered nurses who traditionally provide assessment and complex or invasive interventions (skilled treatments), education, and referral.
- **N3c.** **Homemaking services** — Services that traditionally include IADL support, usually in the form of housekeeping services, shopping, and meal preparation.
- **N3d.** **Meals** — Prepared meals that are delivered to the person for immediate or later consumption (for example, meals-on-wheels).
- **N3e.** **Physical therapy** — Therapy services that are provided or directly supervised by a qualified physical therapist. A qualified physical therapy assistant may provide therapy, but may not supervise others giving therapy.
- **N3f.** **Occupational therapy** — Therapy services that are provided or directly supervised by a qualified occupational therapist. A qualified occupational therapy assistant may provide therapy, but may not supervise others giving therapy.
- **N3g.** **Speech-language pathology and audiology services** — Services provided by a qualified speech-language pathologist. Services may involve assessment of swallowing ability or hearing ability, swallowing therapy, speech therapy, communication therapy, providing hearing appliances, and education.
- **N3h.** **Psychological therapy** — Therapy given by a licensed mental health professional, such as a psychiatrist, psychologist, psychiatric nurse, or psychiatric social worker.

Process	Ask the person or helper(s) about the agencies involved with care, the nature of the relationship, and the amount of time spent in providing care or care management.

Coding   Code the number of days in the first column (maximum = 7) and the number of minutes in the second column, one digit per box. Based on the information available to you, select the best category for the type of support provided. **Do not code twice for the same service.** If the agency did not provide a particular form of care, enter **"0"** in the appropriate box(es). Do not code for care that the person received privately (i.e., from sources other than the agency).

Example of How to Code Formal Care

In the last 7 days the person received from the home care agency 2 hours of home health aide service on 3 days to assist with bathing; visiting nurse service once for 1 hour and 15 minutes to review medications with the client and family and do a physical assessment; and a homemaker once for 3½ hours for cleaning. In addition, the person had a volunteer from the "visiting volunteer" agency for 1 hour on each of 3 days, as well as a privately paid speech therapist on 2 days, for 4½ hours total.

Code as follows:

	# of Days in Last Week	Total Minutes in Last Week		
N3a. Home health aide	3	3	6	0
N3b. Home nurse	1	0	7	5
N3c. Homemaking services	1	2	1	0
N3d. Meals	0	0	0	0
N3e. Physical therapy	0	0	0	0
N3f. Occupational therapy	0	0	0	0
N3g. Speech-language pathology and audiology services	0	0	0	0
N3h. Psychological therapy	0	0	0	0

N4. Hospital Use, Emergency Room Use, Physician Visit in Last 90 Days (or Since Last Assessment if Less Than 90 Days Ago)

N4a. Inpatient acute hospital with overnight stay

Intent   To record how many times the person was admitted to the hospital with an overnight stay in the last 90 days (or since the last assessment, if the person was assessed less than 90 days ago).

Definition   The person was formally admitted as an inpatient (by physician's order), and stayed over 1 or more nights. It does not include admissions for day surgery, outpatient services, etc.

Process   Review prior hospitalizations with the person and family. If available, review the clinical record. Sometimes transmittal or billing records from recent hospital admissions are available.

Coding	Enter the number of hospital admissions in the box. Enter **"0"** in both boxes if no hospital admissions occurred in the last 90 days. If the code is a single digit, use a leading zero to fill in the first box.
N4b.	**Emergency room visit (not counting overnight stay)**
Intent	To record if during the last 90 days (or since the last assessment, if the person was assessed less than 90 days ago) the person visited a hospital emergency room (ER) for treatment or evaluation, not including any ER visits that were accompanied by an overnight hospital stay.
Process	Ask the person and family and review transmittal records if available.
Coding	Enter the number of ER visits in the last 90 days (or since last assessment). Enter **"0"** in both boxes if no ER visits occurred. Do not include instances in which the person was admitted to the hospital for an overnight stay after being seen in the ER. If the code is a single digit, use a leading zero to fill in the first box.
N4c.	**Physician visit (or authorized assistant or practitioner)**
Intent	To record the person's visits to (or from) doctors and authorized assistants or practitioners during the last 90 days (or since the last assessment, if the person was assessed less than 90 days ago).
Definition	A visit to a medical provider's office or clinic by the person, or a medical provider's visit to the person's home. This item includes a very broad spectrum of medical providers and specialists—for example, MDs or osteopaths, who may be either the primary physician or consultant(s); authorized physician's assistants; or nurse-practitioners.
Coding	Enter the number of visits with a physician or authorized assistant or practitioner during the last 90 days (or since the last assessment, if the person was assessed less than 90 days ago). If there were no such visits, enter **"0"** in both boxes. If the code is a single digit, use a leading zero to fill in the first box.

N5. Physically Restrained

Definition	For example, the person's limbs were restrained; the person used bed rails; or the person was restrained to the chair when sitting.
Coding	Indicate whether the person was physically restrained in the last 3 days, regardless of stated intent of restraint. 0. No 1. Yes

Section O

Responsibility

01. **Legal Guardian [Country Specific]**

NOTE: If not in the USA, please consult your addendum.

Intent   To determine if the person has a court-appointed representative.

Definition   A person legally responsible for the person being assessed.

Coding   Code for the appropriate response.

    0. No

    1. Yes

Section P

Social Supports

P1. Two Key Informal Helpers

Intent
To assess the person's informal caregiver support system. This is different from a formal relationship that the person may have with a home care agency.

Definitions
Helper 1 — This is the primary informal helper, who may be a family member, friend, or neighbor, but not a paid service provider. It is not required that the caregiver actually live with the person, but he or she must visit regularly and respond to the person's needs. This is the individual the person views as most helpful to him or her (that is, who can most be relied on).

Helper 2 — This is the secondary informal helper, the individual whom, after the primary helper, the person most relies on to help or give advice and counsel when needed.

Process
Ask the person to identify his or her two most important informal helpers. Shape the questions with specific statements: "Who helps you shop?" "Who helps with cleaning around the house?" "Who helps you with your meals, bathing, dressing, etc.?" "Who helps you pay your bills?" "Who drives you when you need a ride?" If the person does not currently have a "helper", ask if there is someone who "would help" if needed; the person may be able to identify several people. If the person is not able to understand or respond to questions, or gives responses that are unclear, evasive, or untrue (for example, refers to her husband when you know the husband is deceased), review any agency documentation or ask informal helpers if available.

It is important to understand that some helpers may not be described as such by the person. They do things consistent with "expected" social relationships—it is what the person expects a daughter or wife to "do". Thus, it is useful to focus the person's attention on who provides needed assistance or support, rather than using the label "caregiver".

P1a. Relationship to person

Definition
This refers to the nature of the relationship(s) between the person and the informal helper(s). Consider the quality of the relationship, not simply as the relationship is defined by the law or social customs. For example, if the person has a nonrelated "partner" and it appears (and they consider) that the relationship is "like a marriage" but is not legally recognized, code as **"3"** for "Partner/significant other".

Process
Ask the person and the helper (where available) about the nature of their relationship. Validate the significance of their relationship, as they define it.

Coding
For both columns (Helper 1 and Helper 2), code with the category below that best describes the relationship. If only one informal helper has been identified for the person, enter **"9"** in the column for Helper 2.

1. Child or child-in-law
2. Spouse
3. Partner/significant other
4. Parent/guardian
5. Sibling
6. Other relative
7. Friend
8. Neighbor
9. No informal helper

P1b.	**Lives with person**
Intent	To assess whether the person lives with the informal helper(s), and the duration of the living arrangement.
Definition	An informal helper is said to live with the person if the person and helper share the same space (house, apartment/flat). This does not include living in an adjacent or neighboring apartment/flat/house.
Coding	For both columns (Helper 1 and Helper 2), use the following codes.

0. No
1. Yes, 6 months or less
2. Yes, more than 6 months
8. No informal helper

Areas of Informal Help During the Last 3 Days

P1c.	**IADL help**
Definition	Includes activities such as meal preparation, ordinary housework, managing finances or medications, phone use, shopping, and transportation.
Process	Ask the person and informal helper(s), when available, if support is given in meal preparation, ordinary housework, managing finances or medications, phone use, shopping, and transportation. Such support from the helper(s) can range from doing light housework only to doing all of the shopping and housework.
Coding	For each column (Helper 1 and Helper 2), code "Yes" if the helper is assisting the person with IADLs.

0. No
1. Yes
8. No informal helper

P1d.	ADL help
Definition	Includes activities such as bed mobility, transferring, walking, dressing, eating, toilet use, personal hygiene, and bathing.
Process	Ask the person and informal helper(s), when available, if support is given in ADL areas such as bed mobility, transferring, walking, dressing, eating, toilet use, personal hygiene, and bathing. Such support from the helper(s) can range from "being there just in case" (to provide reassurance or ensure safety) to providing complete ADL care.
Coding	For each column (Helper 1 and Helper 2), code "Yes" if the helper is assisting the person with ADLs. 0. No 1. Yes 8. **No informal helper**

P2. Informal Helper Status

Intent	To assess the reserves of the informal caregiver support system.
Definitions	**P2a. Informal helper(s) is (are) unable to continue in caring activities** — For example, a decline in the health of a caregiver/helper makes it difficult to continue. The caregiver, person, or assessor believes that the caregiver(s) is (are) not able to continue in caring activities. This can be for any reason—for example, lack of desire to continue; geographical inaccessibility; other competing requirements, such as child care or work requirements; or personal health issues. **P2b. Primary informal helper expresses feelings of distress, anger, or depression** — Primary caregiver expresses, by any means, that he or she is distressed, angry, depressed, or in conflict because of caring for the person. **P2c. Family or close friends report feeling overwhelmed by person's illness** — Family members or close friends of the person indicate that they are having trouble handling the illness. They may vocalize their feelings of being "overwhelmed" or "stressed out."
Process	Ask the informal caregiver(s) and person separately about the ability of the caregiver(s) to continue providing care. For these items, you need to consider the current situation and also project future needs. The caregiver may be willing and able to continue, but the person may believe him- or herself to be a burden and state that the caregiver cannot continue. Take this information into consideration and use your clinical judgment to make the assessment. This is a sensitive issue and should be handled carefully. Listen carefully to what is being said.
Coding	0. No 1. Yes

P3. Hours of Informal Care and Active Monitoring During Last 3 Days

Intent To capture the number of hours informal helpers spent assisting the person in instrumental and personal activities of daily living, including active monitoring by looking in on the person, over the last 3 days.

Definitions **Informal care** — This means care by all the family, friends, neighbors, and so forth who provide assistance to the person, including but not limited to the primary caregiver (Helper 1).

Instrumental activities of daily living (IADLs) — These include meal preparation, housework, managing finances, etc.

Personal activities of daily living (ADLs)) — These include mobility in bed, dressing, toilet use, etc.

Process Consult with the person about hours of care. Confirm information with the primary caregiver.

Coding Record the total amount of help the person received from family, friends, or neighbors over the last 3 days. For example, if family members, friends, and neighbors provided 120 minutes (2 hours) each day, the total number of hours for help received during the last 3 days is 6. If more than one individual provided help, at the same time or at different times, add up the hours for each individual—for example, if two neighbors spent an hour together doing housecleaning for the person, this would count as 2 hours.

Round minutes to the nearest hour. For example, 12 hours and 45 minutes should be coded as 13 hours.

If the person did not receive any informal care during the last 3 days, enter "0" in all three boxes. If the number of hours is single-digit or double-digit, use leading zero(s) to fill in the first box(es).

P4. Strong and Supportive Relationship with Family

Definition The person indicates he or she has a supportive relationship with family members. The person may feel able to "rely on" family members. Family members may be actively involved in the person's physical care, maintaining the household, managing finances, or helping the person make medical decisions.

Coding 0. No
1. Yes

Section Q

Environmental Assessment

Q1.		**Home Environment**
Intent		To determine if the home environment is hazardous or uninhabitable.
Definitions	Q1a.	**Disrepair of the home** — For example, hazardous clutter; inadequate or no lighting in living room, sleeping room, kitchen, toilet, or corridors; holes in floor; or leaking pipes.
	Q1b.	**Squalid condition** — For example, extremely dirty. There may be dried urine, feces, or dried food on the floor, or infestation by insects or vermin (such as mice or rats). For an environment to be coded as "squalid", the condition must be much more deteriorated than "usual" clutter and household dust and dirt accumulated over a week or so.
	Q1c.	**Inadequate heating or cooling** — Heating and cooling systems may be inadequate (for example, too hot in summer or too cold in winter) or inappropriate (for example, too cold in summer or too hot in winter and not controllable by the person or caregiver).
	Q1d.	**Lack of personal safety** — For example, fear of violence, a safety problem in going to the mailbox or visiting neighbors, or heavy traffic in the street. The person is (or feels) at risk for violence within or immediately outside of his or her home. This can include a real or perceived risk of someone breaking into the home, or of being attacked while getting mail or when leaving or returning home.
	Q1e.	**Limited access to home or rooms in home** — For example, the person has difficulty entering or leaving the home, is unable to climb stairs, or has difficulty maneuvering within rooms. This item includes physical problems with the building that limit access—for example, the person lives on the second floor and must enter or leave on unstable outside stairs, or the person lives in a multistory building in which the elevator is often broken, or in which stairs do not have the needed railings.
Process		Ask the person (or family member) for permission to walk through the home. Look for evidence of the problem areas noted in this section. Talk to the person (and family member if necessary) about any areas that you cannot assess yourself through visual inspection.

Q2.		**Lives in Apartment or House Re-Engineered Accessible for Persons with Disabilities**
Coding		0. No
		1. Yes

Q3.		**Outside Environment**

Definitions	**Q3a. Availability of emergency assistance** — For example, telephone, alarm response system. The person indicates that he or she has access to emergency assistance. This could be by means of a telephone, or speed dialing option on the telephone, or an emergency response system.
	Q3b. Accessibility to grocery store without assistance — The person is able to go to the grocery store and make purchases without assistance. The person may travel to the grocery store by walking, driving or riding a car, or riding in a bus, trolley, subway or cab.
	Q3c. Availability of home delivery of groceries — Code regardless of whether or not the person is using such a service at the present time.
Coding	0. No
	1. Yes

Q4.		**Finances**

Intent	To determine if limited funds prevented the person from receiving required medical and environmental support.
Definition	**Limited funds** — Because of insufficient funds during the last 30 days, the person made trade-offs among purchasing any of the following: adequate food, shelter, clothing; prescribed medications; sufficient home heat or cooling; necessary health care.
Process	Ask the person, or caregiver, if prescribed medications, sufficient home heat (electricity, gas), necessary medical care, or adequate food were not obtained due to insufficient funds. Asking financial questions can be a sensitive area. Questioning must be sensitive and respectful to the person.
Coding	Code for the most appropriate category.
	0. No
	1. Yes

Section R

Discharge Potential and Overall Status

R1. **One or More Care Goals Met in the Last 90 Days (or Since Last Assessment if Less Than 90 Days Ago)**

Intent — To identify if any of the person's treatment goals, established by the person or members of the care team (for example, by nurses, social workers, therapists, or medical doctors), have been achieved in the last 90 days (or since the last assessment, if that was less than 90 days ago).

Process — Confer with the person and clinical professionals; review any clinical documentation. Question the person to determine his or her perception regarding an improvement in function or return to health. Keep in mind that discussions with professionals may be biased by payment category (for example, fee for service) or the nature of the care (for example, open-ended maintenance program).

Coding — Code the appropriate response.

0. No

1. Yes

R2. **Overall Self-Sufficiency Has Changed Significantly as Compared to Status of 90 Days Ago (or Since Last Assessment if Less Than 90 Days Ago)**

Intent — To monitor the person's overall self-sufficiency in the community over time. If this is the person's first assessment, include changes during the period prior to admission to the service agency.

Definition — **Overall self-sufficiency** — Includes self-care performance and support, continence patterns, involvement patterns, use of treatments, etc.

Process — Discuss with the person. If available, review clinical records, transmittal records (if new admission or readmission), previous assessments (if this is a reassessment), and any care plan notes if available. If necessary, discuss with a family member or caregiver.

Coding — Record the number corresponding to the most correct response. If the score is "0" or "1", you should then proceed directly to Section S; if the score is "3", complete the remainder of Section R before moving on to Section S.

0. Improved (Skip to Section S)

1. No change (Skip to Section S)

2. Deteriorated

> ### Examples of How to Code for Changes in Self-Sufficiency
>
> Mrs. T has had Alzheimer's disease for several years. In the past 4 months her overall condition has generally improved. Although her cognitive function has remained unchanged, her mood is improved. She seems happier and less agitated, sleeps more soundly at night, and is more socially involved with her husband and neighbors. **Code "0" for "Improved".**
>
> Mr. D also has a several-year history of Alzheimer's disease. Although for the past year he was quite dependent on others in many areas, he was able to put on his own clothes, walk, and eat with supervision until recently. In the past 90 days he has become more dependent in walking. He can no longer walk without someone holding his arm. Additionally, he fell 2 weeks ago and has been unable to learn how to use a walker on his own. He sits until someone gets the walker and accompanies him as he leaves his apartment. He is fearful of falling again. **Code "2" for "Deteriorated".**

NOTE: Code the following three items if the person "deteriorated" in the last 90 days (or since the last assessment, if less than 90 days have passed since then). Otherwise, skip these items and go directly to Section S.

R3. Number of 10 ADL Areas in Which Person Was Independent Prior to Deterioration

Definition 10 ADL areas — See Item G2 for the complete list of activities of daily living (ADLs), beginning with "Bathing" (G2a) and ending with "Eating" (G2j).

Coding Enter the number of ADLs in which the person was independent before the deterioration that occurred during the assessment period. If the number is a single digit, use a leading zero to fill in the first box.

R4. Number of 8 IADL Performance Areas in Which Person Was Independent Prior to Deterioration

Definition 8 IADL areas — See Item G1 for the complete list of instrumental activities of daily living (IADLs), beginning with "Meal preparation" (G1a) and ending with "Transportation" (G1h).

Coding Enter the number of IADLs in which the person was independent before the deterioration that occurred during the assessment period.

R5. Time of Onset of the Precipitating Event or Problem Related to Deterioration

Coding Select the most appropriate code from the following list.

0. **Within last 7 days**
1. **8 to 14 days ago**
2. **15 to 30 days ago**
3. **31 to 60 days ago**
4. **More than 60 days ago**
8. **No clear precipitating event**

Section S

Discharge

NOTE: Complete this section at discharge only.

S1. **Last Day of Stay**

Coding

Enter the date of the last day of the person's participation in your home care agency, home services, or other health care services. If the month or day contains only a single digit, fill the first box with a "0".

2	0	0	5		1	2		1	7

Year — Month — Day

S2. **Residential/Living Status after Discharge**

Intent

To document the person's living arrangement after his or her discharge from the home care program.

Definitions

1. **Private home/apartment/rented room** — Any house, condominium, apartment, or room in the community, whether owned or rented by the person or another party. Also included in this category are retirement communities or independent housing for older adults or the disabled.

2. **Board and care or assisted living** — A noninstitutional community residential setting that integrates a shared living environment with varying degrees of supportive services of the following types: supervision, home health, homemaker, personal care, meal service, transportation, etc.

3. **Assisted living or semi-independent living** — Other noninstitutional community residential setting that integrates a shared living environment with varying degrees of supportive services of the following types: supervision, home health, homemaker, personal care, meal service, transportation, etc.

4. **Mental health residence** — For example, a psychiatric group home. A residential setting for adults with mental health problems who need supervision and limited services (meals, housekeeping).

5. **Group home for persons with physical disability** — A setting that provides services to persons with physical disabilities. Typically, persons live in group settings with 24-hour staff presence. Individuals are encouraged to be as independent and active as possible.

6. **Setting for persons with intellectual disability** — A setting that provides services to persons with intellectual disabilities. Typically, persons live in group settings with 24-hour staff presence, but are encouraged to be as independent and active as possible.

7. **Psychiatric hospital or unit** — A hospital that focuses on the diagnosis and treatment of psychiatric disorders and which is separate from other inpatient facilities, such as an acute care, rehabilitation, or chronic care hospital. A

psychiatric unit is a care unit, located in a general hospital, which is dedicated to the diagnosis and treatment of psychiatric disorders.

8. **Homeless (with or without shelter)** — A homeless person does not have a fixed residence (a house, apartment, room, or place to stay on a regular basis). The person may live on the streets, or outside in wooded or open areas. The person may sleep in cars, abandoned buildings, under bridges, etc. Persons who are homeless may or may not take advantage of existing homeless shelters.

9. **Long-term care facility (nursing home)** — A licensed health care facility that provides 24-hour skilled or intermediate-level nursing care.

10. **Rehabilitation hospital/unit** — A licensed rehabilitation hospital that focuses on the physical and occupational rehabilitation of individuals who have experienced disease or injury with subsequent decline in physical function. A rehabilitation unit is located within an acute care hospital and focuses on the acute rehabilitation of individuals who have experienced disease or injury with a subsequent decline in physical function.

11. **Hospice facility/palliative care unit** — A hospice facility (or unit within a facility providing more general care) provides care to persons who have a terminal illness with a prognosis of less than 6 months to live as certified by a physician. The goal of hospice care is to provide comfort and quality of life while assisting the person and family. Palliative care is the care of persons whose diseases are not responsive to curative treatments. It targets pain and symptom relief, without precluding use of life-prolonging treatments. Palliative care is often provided from the time a person is diagnosed with a life-threatening illness.

12. **Acute care hospital** — A facility licensed as an acute care hospital that focuses primarily on the diagnosis and treatment of acute medical disorders.

13. **Correctional facility** — Any jail, penitentiary, or halfway house operated by a local, state, or federal government to care for and house persons who have been sentenced to incarceration by a criminal court.

14. **Other** — Any other type of setting not listed above.

15. **Deceased** — The person is no longer alive.

Process   Ask the person or family if you are unsure of where the person will be living.

Coding   Choose only one answer and enter the appropriate code in the boxes provided. If the code is a single digit, leave the first box blank.

Section T

Assessment Information

T1. **Signature of Person Coordinating/Completing the Assessment**

Intent
The Assessment Coordinator (who will usually be the sole assessor in the home care environment) signs and certifies that the assessment is complete.

Coding
The Assessment Coordinator signs his or her name on line 1 and then puts the date that he or she signed the assessment as complete in box 2. This date can differ from the Assessment Reference Date (see Item A9). If the month or day is a single digit, enter a "0" in the first box.

1. **Signature**

2. **Date assessment signed as complete**

2	0	0	6		0	5		1	4
Year					Month			Day	

List of Abbreviations

AC	Acute Care
ADL	Activities of Daily Living
AL	Assisted Living
ATC	anatomical therapeutic chemical
BUN	blood urea nitrogen
CA	Contact Assessment
CAPs	Clinical Assessment Protocols
CF	Mental Health for Correctional Facilities
CHA	Community Health Assessment
CMH	Community Mental Health
CVA	cerebrovascular accident
ESP	Emergency Screener for Psychiatry
GI	gastrointestinal
GU	genitourinary
HC	Home Care
IADL	Instrumental Activities of Daily Living
ICD-CM	International Classification of Diseases, Clinical Modification
ID	Intellectual Disability
LTCF	Long-Term Care Facilities
MDS	Minimum Data Set
MH	Mental Health
NDC	National Drug Code
PAC	Post-Acute Care
PC	Palliative Care
PRN	pro re nata ("as needed")
QOL	Self-Report Quality of Life
RAI	Resident Assessment Instrument
RUGs	Resource Utilization Groups
TENS	transcutaneous electrical nerve stimulation
WELL	Wellness

HC interRAI™ Home Care (HC) Assessment Form 1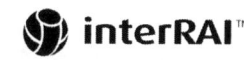
[CODE FOR LAST 3 DAYS, UNLESS OTHERWISE SPECIFIED]

SECTION A. Identification Information

1. **NAME**
   a. (First)   b. (Middle Initial)   c. (Last)   d. (Jr/Sr)

2. **GENDER**
   1. Male   2. Female

3. **BIRTHDATE**
   Year — Month — Day

4. **MARITAL STATUS**
   1 Never married
   2 Married
   3 Partner / Significant other
   4 Widowed
   5 Separated
   6 Divorced

5. **NATIONAL NUMERIC IDENTIFIER [EXAMPLE — USA]**
   a. Social Security number
   b. Medicare number (or comparable railroad insurance number)
   c. Medicaid number [Note: "+" if pending, "N" if not a Medicaid recipient]

6. **FACILITY / AGENCY PROVIDER NUMBER**

7. **CURRENT PAYMENT SOURCES [EXAMPLE — USA]**
   [Note: Billing Office to indicate]
   0 No   1 Yes
   a. Medicaid
   b. Medicare
   c. Self or family pays for full cost
   d. Medicare with Medicaid co-payment
   e. Private insurance
   f. Other per diem

8. **REASON FOR ASSESSMENT**
   1 First assessment
   2 Routine reassessment
   3 Return assessment
   4 Significant change in status reassessment
   5 Discharge assessment, covers last 3 days of service
   6 Discharge tracking only
   7 Other—e.g., research

9. **ASSESSMENT REFERENCE DATE**
   20__ — __ — __
   Year   Month   Day

10. **PERSON'S EXPRESSED GOALS OF CARE**
    Enter primary goal in boxes at bottom

11. **POSTAL / ZIP CODE OF USUAL LIVING ARRANGEMENT [EXAMPLE — USA]**

12. **RESIDENTIAL / LIVING STATUS AT TIME OF ASSESSMENT**
    1 Private home / apartment / rented room
    2 Board and care
    3 Assisted living or semi-independent living
    4 Mental health residence—e.g., psychiatric group home
    5 Group home for persons with physical disability
    6 Setting for persons with intellectual disability
    7 Psychiatric hospital or unit
    8 Homeless (with or without shelter)
    9 Long-term care facility (nursing home)
    10 Rehabilitation hospital / unit
    11 Hospice facility / palliative care unit
    12 Acute care hospital
    13 Correctional facility
    14 Other

13. **LIVING ARRANGEMENT**
    a. Lives
       1 Alone
       2 With spouse / partner only
       3 With spouse / partner and other(s)
       4 With child (not spouse / partner)
       5 With parent(s) or guardian(s)
       6 With sibling(s)
       7 With other relative(s)
       8 With non-relative(s)
    b. As compared to 90 DAYS AGO (or since last assessment), person now lives with someone new—e.g., moved in with another person, other moved in
       0 No   1 Yes
    c. Person or relative feels that the person would be better off living elsewhere
       0 No
       1 Yes, other community residence
       2 Yes, institution

14. **TIME SINCE LAST HOSPITAL STAY**
    Code for most recent instance in LAST 90 DAYS
    0 No hospitalization within 90 days
    1 31 to 90 days ago
    2 15 to 30 days ago
    3 8 to 14 days ago
    4 In the last 7 days
    5 Now in hospital

SECTION B. Intake and Initial History

[Note: Complete at Admission/First Assessment only]

1. **DATE CASE OPENED (this agency)**
   20__ — __ — __
   Year   Month   Day

2. **ETHNICITY AND RACE [EXAMPLE — USA]**
   0 No   1 Yes
   ETHNICITY
   a. Hispanic or Latino
   RACE
   b. American Indian or Alaska Native
   c. Asian
   d. Black or African American
   e. Native Hawaiian or other Pacific Islander
   f. White

3. **PRIMARY LANGUAGE [EXAMPLE — USA]**
   1 English
   2 Spanish
   3 French
   4 Other

4. **RESIDENTIAL HISTORY OVER LAST 5 YEARS**
   Code for all settings person lived in during 5 YEARS prior to date case opened (Item B1)
   0 No   1 Yes
   a. Long-term care facility—e.g., nursing home
   b. Board and care home, assisted living
   c. Mental health residence—e.g., psychiatric group home
   d. Psychiatric hospital or unit
   e. Setting for persons with intellectual disability

© interRAI 1994, 1996, 1997, 1999, 2002, 2005, 2006, 2009 (9.1) [UPDATED MDS-HC 2.0] www.interRAI.org   ISBN: 978-1-936065-01-1

HC interRAI™ Home Care (HC) Assessment Form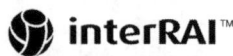

SECTION C. Cognition

1. **COGNITIVE SKILLS FOR DAILY DECISION MAKING**
   Making decisions regarding tasks of daily life—e.g., when to get up or have meals, which clothes to wear or activities to do
   - **0 Independent**—Decisions consistent, reasonable, and safe
   - **1 Modified independence**—Some difficulty in new situations only
   - **2 Minimally impaired**—In specific recurring situations, decisions become poor or unsafe; cues / supervision necessary at those times
   - **3 Moderately impaired**—Decisions consistently poor or unsafe; cues / supervision required at all times
   - **4 Severely impaired**—Never or rarely makes decisions
   - **5 No discernable consciousness, coma [Skip to Section G]**

2. **MEMORY / RECALL ABILITY**
   Code for recall of what was learned or known
   - **0** Yes, memory OK **1** Memory problem
   - a. **Short-term memory OK**—Seems / appears to recall after 5 minutes
   - b. **Procedural memory OK**—Can perform all or almost all steps in a multitask sequence without cues
   - c. **Situational memory OK**—Both: recognizes caregivers' names / faces frequently encountered AND knows location of places regularly visited (bedroom, dining room, activity room, therapy room)

3. **PERIODIC DISORDERED THINKING OR AWARENESS**
   [Note: Accurate assessment requires conversations with staff, family or others who have direct knowledge of the person's behavior over this time]
   - **0** Behavior not present
   - **1** Behavior present, consistent with usual functioning
   - **2** Behavior present, appears different from usual functioning (e.g., new onset or worsening; different from a few weeks ago)
   - a. **Easily distracted**—e.g., episodes of difficulty paying attention; gets sidetracked
   - b. **Episodes of disorganized speech**—e.g., speech is nonsensical, irrelevant, or rambling from subject to subject; loses train of thought
   - c. **Mental function varies over the course of the day**—e.g., sometimes better, sometimes worse

4. **ACUTE CHANGE IN MENTAL STATUS FROM PERSON'S USUAL FUNCTIONING**—e.g., restlessness, lethargy, difficult to arouse, altered environmental perception
   - **0** No **1** Yes

5. **CHANGE IN DECISION MAKING AS COMPARED TO 90 DAYS AGO (OR SINCE LAST ASSESSMENT)**
   - **0** Improved **2** Declined
   - **1** No change **8** Uncertain

SECTION D. Communication and Vision

1. **MAKING SELF UNDERSTOOD (Expression)**
   Expressing information content—both verbal and non-verbal
   - **0 Understood**—Expresses ideas without difficulty
   - **1 Usually understood**—Difficulty finding words or finishing thoughts BUT if given time, little or no prompting required
   - **2 Often understood**—Difficulty finding words or finishing thoughts AND prompting usually required
   - **3 Sometimes understood**—Ability is limited to making concrete requests
   - **4 Rarely or never understood**

2. **ABILITY TO UNDERSTAND OTHERS (Comprehension)**
   Understanding verbal information content (however able; with hearing appliance normally used)
   - **0 Understands**—Clear comprehension
   - **1 Usually understands**—Misses some part / intent of message BUT comprehends most conversation
   - **2 Often understands**—Misses some part / intent of message BUT with repetition or explanation can often comprehend conversation
   - **3 Sometimes understands**—Responds adequately to simple, direct communication only
   - **4 Rarely or never understands**

3. **HEARING**
   Ability to hear (with hearing appliance normally used)
   - **0 Adequate**—No difficulty in normal conversation, social interaction, listening to TV
   - **1 Minimal difficulty**—Difficulty in some environments (e.g., when person speaks softly or is more than 6 feet [2 meters] away)
   - **2 Moderate difficulty**—Problem hearing normal conversation, requires quiet setting to hear well
   - **3 Severe difficulty**—Difficulty in all situations (e.g., speaker has to talk loudly or speak very slowly; or person reports that all speech is mumbled)
   - **4 No hearing**

4. **VISION**
   Ability to see in adequate light (with glasses or with other visual appliance normally used)
   - **0 Adequate**—Sees fine detail, including regular print in newspapers/books
   - **1 Minimal difficulty**—Sees large print, but not regular print in newspapers/books
   - **2 Moderate difficulty**—Limited vision; not able to see newspaper headlines, but can identify objects
   - **3 Severe difficulty**—Object identification in question, but eyes appear to follow objects; sees only light, colors, shapes
   - **4 No vision**

SECTION E. Mood and Behavior

1. **INDICATORS OF POSSIBLE DEPRESSED, ANXIOUS, OR SAD MOOD**
   Code for indicators observed in last 3 days, irrespective of the assumed cause [Note: Whenever possible, ask person]
   - **0** Not present
   - **1** Present but not exhibited in last 3 days
   - **2** Exhibited on 1–2 of last 3 days
   - **3** Exhibited daily in last 3 days
   - a. **Made negative statements**—e.g., "Nothing matters"; "Would rather be dead"; "What's the use"; "Regret having lived so long"; "Let me die"
   - b. **Persistent anger with self or others**—e.g., easily annoyed, anger at care received
   - c. **Expressions, including non-verbal, of what appear to be unrealistic fears**—e.g., fear of being abandoned, being left alone, being with others; intense fear of specific objects or situations
   - d. **Repetitive health complaints**—e.g., persistently seeks medical attention, incessant concern with body functions
   - e. **Repetitive anxious complaints/concerns (non-health related)**—e.g., persistently seeks attention/reassurance regarding schedules, meals, laundry, clothing, relationships
   - f. **Sad, pained, or worried facial expressions**—e.g., furrowed brow, constant frowning
   - g. **Crying, tearfulness**
   - h. **Recurrent statements that something terrible is about to happen**—e.g., believes he or she is about to die, have a heart attack
   - i. **Withdrawal from activities of interest**—e.g., long-standing activities, being with family / friends
   - j. **Reduced social interactions**
   - k. **Expressions, including non-verbal, of a lack of pleasure in life (anhedonia)**—e.g., "I don't enjoy anything anymore"

2. **SELF-REPORTED MOOD**
   - **0** Not in last 3 days
   - **1** Not in last 3 days, but often feels that way
   - **2** In 1–2 of last 3 days
   - **3** Daily in the last 3 days
   - **8** Person could not (would not) respond
   Ask: "In the last 3 days, how often have you felt..."
   - a. **Little interest or pleasure in things you normally enjoy?**
   - b. **Anxious, restless, or uneasy?**
   - c. **Sad, depressed, or hopeless?**

3. BEHAVIOR SYMPTOMS
Code for indicators observed, irrespective of the assumed cause

- **0** Not Present
- **1** Present but not exhibited in last 3 days
- **2** Exhibited on 1–2 of last 3 days
- **3** Exhibited daily in last 3 days

a. **Wandering**—Moved with no rational purpose, seemingly oblivious to needs or safety ☐
b. **Verbal abuse**—e.g., others were threatened, screamed at, cursed at ☐
c. **Physical abuse**—e.g., others were hit, shoved, scratched, sexually abused ☐
d. **Socially inappropriate or disruptive behavior**—e.g., made disruptive sounds or noises, screamed out, smeared or threw food or feces, hoarded, rummaged through other's belongings ☐
e. **Inappropriate public sexual behavior or public disrobing** ☐
f. **Resists care**—e.g., taking medications/injections, ADL assistance, eating ☐

SECTION F. Psychosocial Well-Being

1. SOCIAL RELATIONSHIPS
[Note: Whenever possible, ask person]

- **0** Never
- **1** More than 30 days ago
- **2** 8 to 30 days ago
- **3** 4 to 7 days ago
- **4** In last 3 days
- **8** Unable to determine

a. Participation in social activities of long-standing interest ☐
b. Visit with a long-standing social relation or family member ☐
c. Other interaction with long-standing social relation or family member—e.g., telephone, e-mail ☐
d. Conflict or anger with family or friends ☐
e. Fearful of a family member or close acquaintance ☐
f. Neglected, abused, or mistreated ☐

2. LONELY
Says or indicates that he / she feels lonely ☐

0 No   **1** Yes

3. CHANGE IN SOCIAL ACTIVITIES IN LAST 90 DAYS (OR SINCE LAST ASSESSMENT IF LESS THAN 90 DAYS AGO) ☐
Decline in level of participation in social, religious, occupational, or other preferred activities

IF THERE WAS A DECLINE, person distressed by this fact

- **0** No decline
- **1** Decline, not distressed
- **2** Decline, distressed

4. LENGTH OF TIME ALONE DURING THE DAY (MORNING AND AFTERNOON) ☐

- **0** Less than 1 hour
- **1** 1–2 hours
- **2** More than 2 hours but less than 8 hours
- **3** 8 hours or more

5. MAJOR LIFE STRESSORS IN LAST 90 DAYS—*e.g., episode of severe personal illness; death or severe illness of close family member / friend; loss of home; major loss of income / assets; victim of a crime such as robbery or assault; loss of driving license/car* ☐

0 No   **1** Yes

SECTION G. Functional Status

1. IADL SELF-PERFORMANCE AND CAPACITY
Code for PERFORMANCE in routine activities around the home or in the community during the LAST 3 DAYS

Code for CAPACITY based on presumed ability to carry out activity as independently as possible. This will require "speculation" by the assessor.

- **0** Independent—No help, setup, or supervision
- **1** Setup help only
- **2** Supervision—Oversight / cuing
- **3** Limited assistance—Help on some occasions
- **4** Extensive assistance—Help throughout task, but performs 50% or more of task on own
- **5** Maximal assistance—Help throughout task, but performs less than 50% of task on own
- **6** Total dependence—Full performance by others during entire period
- **8** Activity did not occur—During entire period
  [DO NOT USE THIS CODE IN SCORING CAPACITY]

Performance | Capacity

a. **Meal preparation**—How meals are prepared (e.g., planning meals, assembling ingredients, cooking, setting out food and utensils) ☐ ☐
b. **Ordinary housework**—How ordinary work around the house is performed (e.g., doing dishes, dusting, making bed, tidying up, laundry) ☐ ☐
c. **Managing finances**—How bills are paid, checkbook is balanced, household expenses are budgeted, credit card account is monitored ☐ ☐
d. **Managing medications**—How medications are managed (e.g., remembering to take medicines, opening bottles, taking correct drug dosages, giving injections, applying ointments) ☐ ☐
e. **Phone use**—How telephone calls are made or received (with assistive devices such as large numbers on telephone, amplification as needed) ☐ ☐
f. **Stairs**—How full flight of stairs is managed (12–14 stairs) ☐ ☐
g. **Shopping**—How shopping is performed for food and household items (e.g., selecting items, paying money)—EXCLUDE TRANSPORTATION ☐ ☐
h. **Transportation**—How travels by public transportation (navigating system, paying fare) or driving self (including getting out of house, into and out of vehicles) ☐ ☐

2. ADL SELF-PERFORMANCE
Consider all episodes over 3-day period.

If all episodes are performed at the same level, score ADL at that level.

If any episodes at level 6, and others less dependent, score ADL as a 5.

Otherwise, focus on the three most dependent episodes [or all episodes if performed fewer than 3 times]. If most dependent episode is 1, score ADL as 1. If not, score ADL as least dependent of those episodes in range 2–5.

- **0 Independent**—No physical assistance, setup, or supervision in any episode
- **1 Independent, setup help only**—Article or device provided or placed within reach, no physical assistance or supervision in any episode
- **2 Supervision**—Oversight / cuing
- **3 Limited assistance**—Guided maneuvering of limbs, physical guidance without taking weight
- **4 Extensive assistance**—Weight-bearing support (including lifting limbs) by 1 helper where person still performs 50% or more of subtasks
- **5 Maximal assistance**—Weight-bearing support (including lifting limbs) by 2+ helpers —OR— Weight-bearing support for more than 50% of subtasks
- **6 Total dependence**—Full performance by others during all episodes
- **8 Activity did not occur during entire period**

a. **Bathing**—How takes a full-body bath / shower. Includes how transfers in and out of tub or shower AND how each part of body is bathed: arms, upper and lower legs, chest, abdomen, perineal area — EXCLUDE WASHING OF BACK AND HAIR ☐
b. **Personal hygiene**—How manages personal hygiene, including combing hair, brushing teeth, shaving, applying make-up, washing and drying face and hands — EXCLUDE BATHS AND SHOWERS ☐
c. **Dressing upper body**—How dresses and undresses (street clothes, underwear) above the waist, including prostheses, orthotics, fasteners, pullovers, etc. ☐
d. **Dressing lower body**—How dresses and undresses (street clothes, underwear) from the waist down including prostheses, orthotics, belts, pants, skirts, shoes, fasteners, etc. ☐

HC interRAI™ Home Care (HC) Assessment Form 4   interRAI™

e. **Walking**—How walks between locations on same floor indoors
f. **Locomotion**—How moves between locations on same floor (walking or wheeling). If in wheelchair, self-sufficiency once in chair
g. **Transfer toilet**—How moves on and off toilet or commode
h. **Toilet use**—How uses the toilet room (or commode, bedpan, urinal), cleanses self after toilet use or incontinent episode(s), changes pad, manages ostomy or catheter, adjusts clothes — EXCLUDE TRANSFER ON AND OFF TOILET
i. **Bed mobility**—How moves to and from lying position, turns from side to side, and positions body while in bed
j. **Eating**—How eats and drinks (regardless of skill). Includes intake of nourishment by other means (e.g., tube feeding, total parenteral nutrition)

3. **LOCOMOTION / WALKING**
   a. **Primary mode of locomotion**
      0 Walking, no assistive device
      1 Walking, uses assistive device—e.g., cane, walker, crutch, pushing wheelchair
      2 Wheelchair, scooter
      3 Bedbound
   b. **Timed 4-meter (13-foot) walk**
      Lay out a straight, unobstructed course. Have person stand in still position, feet just touching start line. **Then say: "When I tell you begin to walk at a normal pace (with cane/walker if used). This is not a test of how fast you can walk. Stop when I tell you to stop. Is this clear?"** *Assessor may demonstrate test.* **Then say: "Begin to walk now."** *Start stopwatch (or can count seconds) when first foot falls. End count when foot falls beyond 4-meter mark.* **Then say: "You may stop now."**
      Enter time in seconds, up to 30 seconds
      30 30 or more seconds to walk 4 meters
      77 Stopped before test complete
      88 Refused to do the test
      99 Not tested—e.g., does not walk on own
   c. **Distance walked**—Farthest distance walked at one time without sitting down in the LAST 3 DAYS (with support as needed)
      0 Did not walk
      1 Less than 15 feet (under 5 meters)
      2 15–149 feet (5–49 meters)
      3 150–299 feet (50–99 meters)
      4 300+ feet (100+ meters)
      5 1/2 mile or more (1+ kilometers)
   d. **Distance wheeled self**—Farthest distance wheeled self at one time in the LAST 3 DAYS (includes independent use of motorized wheelchair)
      0 Wheeled by others
      1 Used motorized wheelchair / scooter
      2 Wheeled self less than 15 feet (under 5 meters)
      3 Wheeled self 15–149 feet (5–49 meters)
      4 Wheeled self 150–299 feet (50–99 meters)
      5 Wheeled self 300+ feet (100+ meters)
      8 Did not use wheelchair

4. **ACTIVITY LEVEL**
   a. **Total hours of exercise or physical activity in LAST 3 DAYS**—e.g., walking
      0 None
      1 Less than 1 hour
      2 1–2 hours
      3 3–4 hours
      4 More than 4 hours
   b. **In the LAST 3 DAYS, number of days went out of the house or building in which he/she resides** (no matter how short the period)
      0 No days out
      1 Did not go out in last 3 days, but usually goes out over a 3-day period
      2 1–2 days
      3 3 days

5. **PHYSICAL FUNCTION IMPROVEMENT POTENTIAL**
      0 No   1 Yes
   a. Person believes he / she is capable of improved performance in physical function
   b. Care professional believes person is capable of improved performance in physical function

6. **CHANGE IN ADL STATUS AS COMPARED TO 90 DAYS AGO, OR SINCE LAST ASSESSMENT IF LESS THAN 90 DAYS AGO**
      0 Improved
      1 No change
      2 Declined
      3 Uncertain

7. **DRIVING**
   a. Drove car (vehicle) in the LAST 90 DAYS
      0 No   1 Yes
   b. If drove in LAST 90 DAYS, assessor is aware that someone has suggested that person limits OR stops driving
      0 No, or does not drive   1 Yes

SECTION H. Continence

1. **BLADDER CONTINENCE**
      0 **Continent**—Complete control; DOES NOT USE any type of catheter or other urinary collection device
      1 **Control with any catheter or ostomy** over last 3 days
      2 **Infrequently incontinent**—Not incontinent over last 3 days, but does have incontinent episodes
      3 **Occasionally incontinent**—Less than daily
      4 **Frequently incontinent**—Daily, but some control present
      5 **Incontinent**—No control present
      8 **Did not occur**—No urine output from bladder in last 3 days
2. **URINARY COLLECTION DEVICE [Exclude pads / briefs]**
      0 None
      1 Condom catheter
      2 Indwelling catheter
      3 Cystostomy, nephrostomy, ureterostomy

3. **BOWEL CONTINENCE**
      0 **Continent**—Complete control; DOES NOT USE any type of ostomy device
      1 **Control with ostomy**—Control with ostomy device over last 3 days
      2 **Infrequently incontinent**—Not incontinent over last 3 days, but does have incontinent episodes
      3 **Occasionally incontinent**—Less than daily
      4 **Frequently incontinent**—Daily, but some control present
      5 **Incontinent**—No control present
      8 **Did not occur**—No bowel movement in the last 3 days
4. **PADS OR BRIEFS WORN**
      0 No   1 Yes

SECTION I. Disease Diagnoses

Disease code
      0 Not present
      1 Primary diagnosis/diagnoses for current stay
      2 Diagnosis present, receiving active treatment
      3 Diagnosis present, monitored but no active treatment

1. **DISEASE DIAGNOSES**
   MUSCULOSKELETAL
   a. Hip fracture during last 30 days (or since last assessment if less than 30 days)
   b. Other fracture during last 30 days (or since last assessment if less than 30 days)

   NEUROLOGICAL
   c. Alzheimer's disease
   d. Dementia other than Alzheimer's disease
   e. Hemiplegia
   f. Multiple sclerosis
   g. Paraplegia
   h. Parkinson's disease
   i. Quadriplegia
   j. Stroke / CVA

| HC | interRAI™ Home Care (HC) Assessment Form | 5 |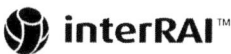

CARDIAC OR PULMONARY
- k. Coronary heart disease
- l. Chronic obstructive pulmonary disease
- m. Congestive heart failure

PSYCHIATRIC
- n. Anxiety
- o. Bipolar disorder
- p. Depression
- q. Schizophrenia

INFECTIONS
- r. Pneumonia
- s. Urinary tract infection in last 30 days

OTHER
- t. Cancer
- u. Diabetes mellitus

2. OTHER DISEASE DIAGNOSES

Diagnosis	Disease Code	ICD code
a.	☐	| | | • | | |
b.	☐	| | | • | | |
c.	☐	| | | • | | |
d.	☐	| | | • | | |
e.	☐	| | | • | | |
f.	☐	| | | • | | |

[Note: Add additional lines as necessary for other disease diagnoses]

SECTION J. Health Conditions

1. FALLS
- **0** No fall in last 90 days
- **1** No fall in last 30 days, but fell 31–90 days ago
- **2** One fall in last 30 days
- **3** Two or more falls in last 30 days

2. RECENT FALLS
[Skip if last assessed more than 30 days ago or if this is first assessment]
- **0** No
- **1** Yes
- **[blank]** Not applicable (first assessment, or more than 30 days since last assessment)

3. PROBLEM FREQUENCY
Code for presence in last 3 days
- **0** Not present
- **1** Present but not exhibited in last 3 days
- **2** Exhibited on 1 of last 3 days
- **3** Exhibited on 2 of last 3 days
- **4** Exhibited daily in last 3 days

BALANCE
- a. Difficult or unable to move self to standing position unassisted
- b. Difficult or unable to turn self around and face the opposite direction when standing
- c. Dizziness
- d. Unsteady gait

CARDIAC OR PULMONARY
- e. Chest pain
- f. Difficulty clearing airway secretions

PSYCHIATRIC
- g. Abnormal thought process—e.g., loosening of associations, blocking, flight of ideas, tangentiality, circumstantiality
- h. Delusions—Fixed false beliefs
- i. Hallucinations—False sensory perceptions

NEUROLOGICAL
- j. Aphasia

GI STATUS
- k. Acid reflux—Regurgitation of acid from stomach to throat
- l. Constipation—No bowel movement in 3 days or difficult passage of hard stool
- m. Diarrhea
- n. Vomiting

SLEEP PROBLEMS
- o. Difficulty falling asleep or staying asleep; waking up too early; restlessness; non-restful sleep
- p. Too much sleep—Excessive amount of sleep that interferes with person's normal functioning

OTHER
- q. Aspiration
- r. Fever
- s. GI or GU bleeding
- t. Hygiene—Unusually poor hygiene, unkempt, disheveled
- u. Peripheral edema

4. DYSPNEA (Shortness of breath)
- **0** Absence of symptom
- **1** Absent at rest, but present when performed moderate activities
- **2** Absent at rest, but present when performed normal day-to-day activities
- **3** Present at rest

5. FATIGUE
Inability to complete normal daily activities—e.g., ADLs, IADLs
- **0 None**
- **1 Minimal**—Diminished energy but completes normal day-to-day activities
- **2 Moderate**—Due to diminished energy, UNABLE TO FINISH normal day-to-day activities
- **3 Severe**—Due to diminished energy, UNABLE TO START SOME normal day-to-day activities
- **4 Unable to commence any normal day-to-day activities**—Due to diminished energy

6. PAIN SYMPTOMS
[Note: Always ask the person about pain frequency, intensity, and control. Observe person and ask others who are in contact with the person.]

- a. **Frequency with which person complains or shows evidence of pain** (including grimacing, teeth clenching, moaning, withdrawal when touched, or other nonverbal signs suggesting pain)
  - **0** No pain
  - **1** Present but not exhibited in last 3 days
  - **2** Exhibited on 1–2 of last 3 days
  - **3** Exhibited daily in last 3 days

- b. **Intensity of highest level of pain present**
  - **0** No pain
  - **1** Mild
  - **2** Moderate
  - **3** Severe
  - **4** Times when pain is horrible or excruciating

- c. **Consistency of pain**
  - **0** No pain
  - **1** Single episode during last 3 days
  - **2** Intermittent
  - **3** Constant

- d. **Breakthrough pain**—Times in LAST 3 DAYS when person experienced sudden, acute flare-ups of pain
  - **0** No   **1** Yes

- e. **Pain control**—Adequacy of current therapeutic regimen to control pain (from person's point of view)
  - **0** No issue of pain
  - **1** Pain intensity acceptable to person; no treatment regimen or change in regimen required
  - **2** Controlled adequately by therapeutic regimen
  - **3** Controlled when therapeutic regimen followed, but not always followed as ordered
  - **4** Therapeutic regimen followed, but pain control not adequate
  - **5** No therapeutic regimen being followed for pain; pain not adequately controlled

7. INSTABILITY OF CONDITIONS
0 No   **1** Yes

     a. Conditions / diseases make cognitive, ADL, mood or behavior patterns unstable (fluctuating, precarious, or deteriorating) ☐
     b. Experiencing an acute episode, or a flare-up of a recurrent or chronic problem ☐
     c. End-stage disease, 6 or fewer months to live ☐

8. SELF-REPORTED HEALTH
Ask: "In general, how would you rate your health?"

     0 Excellent
     1 Good
     2 Fair
     3 Poor
     8 Could not (would not) respond

9. TOBACCO AND ALCOHOL
     a. Smokes tobacco daily ☐
         0 No
         1 Not in last 3 days, but is usually a daily smoker
         2 Yes
     b. Alcohol—Highest number of drinks in any "single sitting" in LAST 14 DAYS ☐
         0 None
         1 1
         2 2–4
         3 5 or more

SECTION K. Oral And Nutritional Status

1. HEIGHT AND WEIGHT [INCHES AND POUNDS — COUNTRY SPECIFIC]
Record (a.) height in inches and (b.) weight in pounds. Base weight on most recent measure in LAST 30 DAYS.

     a. **HT** (in.) ☐☐   b. **WT** (lb.) ☐☐

2. NUTRITIONAL ISSUES
0 No   **1** Yes

     a. Weight loss of 5% or more in LAST 30 DAYS, or 10% or more in LAST 180 DAYS ☐
     b. Dehydrated or BUN / Cre ratio>25 [Ratio, country specific] ☐
     c. Fluid intake less than 1,000 cc per day (less than four 8 oz cups/day) ☐
     d. Fluid output exceeds input ☐

3. MODE OF NUTRITIONAL INTAKE
     0 Normal—Swallows all types of foods
     1 Modified independent—e.g., liquid is sipped, takes limited solid food, need for modification may be unknown
     2 Requires diet modification to swallow solid food—e.g., mechanical diet (e.g., puree, minced, etc.) or only able to ingest specific foods
     3 Requires modification to swallow liquids—e.g., thickened liquids
     4 Can swallow only pureed solids—AND—thickened liquids
     5 Combined oral and parenteral or tube feeding
     6 Nasogastric tube feeding only
     7 Abdominal feeding tube—e.g., PEG tube
     8 Parenteral feeding only—Includes all types of parenteral feedings, such as total parenteral nutrition (TPN)
     9 Activity did not occur—During entire period

4. DENTAL OR ORAL
0 No   **1** Yes

     a. Wears a denture (removable prosthesis) ☐
     b. Has broken, fragmented, loose, or otherwise non-intact natural teeth ☐
     c. Reports having dry mouth ☐
     d. Reports difficulty chewing ☐

SECTION L. Skin Condition

1. MOST SEVERE PRESSURE ULCER ☐
     0 No pressure ulcer
     1 Any area of persistent skin redness
     2 Partial loss of skin layers
     3 Deep craters in the skin
     4 Breaks in skin exposing muscle or bone
     5 Not codeable, e.g., necrotic eschar predominant

2. PRIOR PRESSURE ULCER ☐
     0 No   **1** Yes

3. PRESENCE OF SKIN ULCER OTHER THAN PRESSURE ULCER— ☐
e.g., venous ulcer, arterial ulcer, mixed venous-arterial ulcer, diabetic foot ulcer
     0 No   **1** Yes

4. MAJOR SKIN PROBLEMS—*e.g., lesions, 2nd or 3rd degree burns, healing surgical wounds* ☐
     0 No   **1** Yes

5. SKIN TEARS OR CUTS—*Other than surgery* ☐
     0 No   **1** Yes

6. OTHER SKIN CONDITIONS OR CHANGES IN SKIN CONDITION— ☐
e.g., bruises, rashes, itching, mottling, herpes zoster, intertrigo, eczema
     0 No   **1** Yes

7. FOOT PROBLEMS—*e.g., bunions, hammer toes, overlapping toes, structural problems, infections, ulcers*
     0 No foot problems
     1 Foot problems, no limitation in walking
     2 Foot problems limit walking
     3 Foot problems prevent walking
     4 Foot problems, does not walk for other reasons

SECTION M. Medications

1. LIST OF ALL MEDICATIONS
List all active prescriptions, and any non-prescribed (over-the-counter) medications taken in the LAST 3 DAYS

[Note: Use computerized records if possible; hand enter only when absolutely necessary]

For each drug record:

     a. **Name**
     b. **Dose**—A positive number such as 0.5, 5, 150, 300.
     [Note: Never write a zero by itself after a decimal point (X mg). Always use a zero before a decimal point (0.X mg)]

     c. **Unit**—Code using the following list:

gtts	(Drops)	**mEq**	(Milli-equivalent)	**Puffs**	
gm	(Gram)	**mg**	(Milligram)	**%**	(Percent)
L	(Liters)	**ml**	(Milliliter)	**Units**	
mcg	(Microgram)	**oz**	(Ounce)	**OTH**	(Other)

     d. **Route of administration**—Code using the following list:

PO	(By mouth/oral)	**REC**	(Rectal)	**ET**	(Enteral Tube)
SL	(Sublingual)	**TOP**	(Topical)	**TD**	(Transdermal)
IM	(Intramuscular)	**IH**	(Inhalation)	**EYE**	(Eye)
IV	(Intravenous)	**NAS**	(Nasal)	**OTH**	(Other)
Sub-Q	(Subcutaneous)				

e. **Freq**—Code the number of times per day, week, or month the medication is administered using the following list:

Q1H (Every hour)		**5D**	(5 times daily)
Q2H (Every 2 hours)		**Q2D**	(Every other day)
Q3H (Every 3 hours)		**Q3D**	(Every 3 days)
Q4H (Every 4 hours)		**Weekly**	
Q6H (Every 6 hours)		**2W**	(2 times weekly)
Q8H (Every 8 hours)		**3W**	(3 times weekly)
Daily		**4W**	(4 times weekly)
BED (At bedtime)		**5W**	(5 times weekly)
BID (2 times daily)		**6W**	(6 times weekly)
(includes every 12 hrs)		**1M**	(Monthly)
TID (3 times daily)		**2M**	(Twice every month)
QID (4 times daily)		**OTH**	(Other)

f. **PRN**
  0 No   **1** Yes

g. **Computer-entered drug code**

	a. Name	b. Dose	c. Unit	d. Route	e. Freq.	f. PRN	g. ATC or NDC code
1.							
2.							
3.							
4.							
5.							

[Note: Add additional lines, as necessary, for other drugs taken]
[Abbreviations are Country Specific for Unit, Route, Frequency]

2. **ALLERGY TO ANY DRUG** ☐
   0 No known drug allergies   **1** Yes

3. **ADHERENT WITH MEDICATIONS PRESCRIBED BY PHYSICIAN** ☐
   0 Always adherent
   1 Adherent 80% of time or more
   2 Adherent less than 80% of time, including failure to purchase prescribed medications
   8 No medications prescribed

SECTION N. Treatments and Procedures

1. **PREVENTION**
   0 No   **1** Yes
   a. Blood pressure measured in LAST YEAR
   b. Colonoscopy test in LAST 5 YEARS
   c. Dental exam in LAST YEAR
   d. Eye exam in LAST YEAR
   e. Hearing exam in LAST 2 YEARS
   f. Influenza vaccine in LAST YEAR
   g. Mammogram or breast exam in LAST 2 YEARS (for women)
   h. Pneumovax vaccine in LAST 5 YEARS or after age 65

2. **TREATMENTS AND PROGRAMS RECEIVED OR SCHEDULED IN THE LAST 3 DAYS (OR SINCE LAST ASSESSMENT IF LESS THAN 3 DAYS)**
   0 Not ordered AND did not occur
   1 Ordered, not implemented
   2 1–2 of last 3 days
   3 Daily in last 3 days

   TREATMENTS
   a. Chemotherapy
   b. Dialysis
   c. Infection control—e.g., isolation, quarantine
   d. IV medication
   e. Oxygen therapy
   f. Radiation
   g. Suctioning
   h. Tracheostomy care
   i. Transfusion
   j. Ventilator or respirator
   k. Wound care

   PROGRAMS
   l. Scheduled toileting program
   m. Palliative care program
   n. Turning / repositioning program

3. **FORMAL CARE**
   Days (A) and Total minutes (B) of care in last 7 days
   Extent of care/treatment in LAST 7 DAYS (or since last assessment or admission, if less than 7 days) involving: (A) # of Days   (B) Total Minutes in Last Week
   a. Home health aides
   b. Home nurse
   c. Homemaking services
   d. Meals
   e. Physical therapy
   f. Occupational therapy
   g. Speech-language pathology and audiology services
   h. Psychological therapy (by any licensed mental health professional)

4. **HOSPITAL USE, EMERGENCY ROOM USE, PHYSICIAN VISIT**
   Code for number of times during the LAST 90 DAYS (or since last assessment if LESS THAN 90 DAYS)
   a. Inpatient acute hospital with overnight stay
   b. Emergency room visit (not counting overnight stay)
   c. Physician visit (or authorized assistant or practitioner)

5. **PHYSICALLY RESTRAINED**—Limbs restrained, used bed rails, restrained to chair when sitting
   0 No   **1** Yes

SECTION O. Responsibility

1. **LEGAL GUARDIAN [EXAMPLE — USA]** ☐
   0 No   **1** Yes

interRAI™ Home Care (HC) Assessment Form

SECTION P. Social Supports

1. TWO KEY INFORMAL HELPERS — Helper 1 2
   a. **Relationship to person**
      - 1 Child or child-in-law
      - 2 Spouse
      - 3 Partner / significant other
      - 4 Parent / guardian
      - 5 Sibling
      - 6 Other relative
      - 7 Friend
      - 8 Neighbor
      - 9 No informal helper
   b. **Lives with person** — Helper 1 2
      - 0 No
      - 1 Yes, 6 months or less
      - 2 Yes, more than 6 months
      - 8 No informal helper

   AREAS OF INFORMAL HELP DURING LAST 3 DAYS — Helper 1 2
      - 0 No
      - 1 Yes
      - 8 No informal helper

      c. IADL help
      d. ADL help

2. INFORMAL HELPER STATUS
   - 0 No
   - 1 Yes

   a. Informal helper(s) is unable to continue in caring activities—e.g., decline in health of helper makes it difficult to continue
   b. Primary informal helper expresses feelings of distress, anger, or depression
   c. Family or close friends report feeling overwhelmed by person's illness

3. HOURS OF INFORMAL CARE AND ACTIVE MONITORING DURING LAST 3 DAYS
   For instrumental and personal activities of daily living in the LAST 3 DAYS, indicate the total number of hours of help received from all family, friends, and neighbors

4. STRONG AND SUPPORTIVE RELATIONSHIP WITH FAMILY
   - 0 No
   - 1 Yes

SECTION Q. Environmental Assessment

1. HOME ENVIRONMENT
   Code for any of following that make home environment hazardous or uninhabitable (if temporarily in institution, base assessment on home visit)
   - 0 No
   - 1 Yes

   a. **Disrepair of the home**—e.g., hazardous clutter; inadequate or no lighting in living room, sleeping room, kitchen, toilet, corridors; holes in floor; leaking pipes
   b. **Squalid condition**—e.g., extremely dirty, infestation by rats or bugs
   c. **Inadequate heating or cooling**—e.g., too hot in summer, too cold in winter
   d. **Lack of personal safety**—e.g., fear of violence, safety problem in going to mailbox or visiting neighbors, heavy traffic in street
   e. **Limited access to home or rooms in home**—e.g., difficulty entering or leaving home, unable to climb stairs, difficulty maneuvering within rooms, no railings although needed

2. LIVES IN APARTMENT OR HOUSE RE-ENGINEERED ACCESSIBLE FOR PERSONS WITH DISABILITIES
   - 0 No
   - 1 Yes

3. OUTSIDE ENVIRONMENT
   - 0 No
   - 1 Yes

   a. **Availability of emergency assistance**—e.g., telephone, alarm response system
   b. **Accessibility to grocery store without assistance**
   c. **Availability of home delivery of groceries**

4. FINANCES
   Because of limited funds, during the last 30 days made trade-offs among purchasing any of the following: adequate food, shelter, clothing; prescribed medications; sufficient home heat or cooling; necessary health care
   - 0 No
   - 1 Yes

SECTION R. Discharge Potential and Overall Status

1. ONE OR MORE CARE GOALS MET IN THE LAST 90 DAYS (OR SINCE LAST ASSESSMENT IF LESS THAN 90 DAYS)
   - 0 No
   - 1 Yes

2. OVERALL SELF-SUFFICIENCY HAS CHANGED SIGNIFICANTLY AS COMPARED TO STATUS OF 90 DAYS AGO (OR SINCE LAST ASSESSMENT IF LESS THAN 90 DAYS)
   - 0 Improved   [Skip to Section S]
   - 1 No change [Skip to Section S]
   - 2 Deteriorated

   CODE FOLLOWING THREE ITEMS IF "DETERIORATED" IN LAST 90 DAYS — OTHERWISE SKIP TO SECTION S

3. NUMBER OF 10 ADL AREAS IN WHICH PERSON WAS INDEPENDENT PRIOR TO DETERIORATION

4. NUMBER OF 8 IADL PERFORMANCE AREAS IN WHICH PERSON WAS INDEPENDENT PRIOR TO DETERIORATION

5. TIME OF ONSET OF THE PRECIPITATING EVENT OR PROBLEM RELATED TO DETERIORATION
   - 0 Within last 7 days
   - 1 8 to 14 days ago
   - 2 15 to 30 days ago
   - 3 31 to 60 days ago
   - 4 More than 60 days ago
   - 8 No clear precipitating event

SECTION S. Discharge

[Note: Complete Section S at Discharge only]

1. LAST DAY OF STAY
   2 0 _ _ — _ _ — _ _
   Year   Month   Day

2. RESIDENTIAL / LIVING STATUS AT TIME OF ASSESSMENT
   1 Private home / apartment / rented room
   2 Board and care
   3 Assisted living or semi-independent living
   4 Mental health residence—e.g., psychiatric group home
   5 Group home for persons with physical disability
   6 Setting for persons with intellectual disability
   7 Psychiatric hospital or unit
   8 Homeless (with or without shelter)
   9 Long-term care facility (nursing home)
   10 Rehabilitation hospital / unit
   11 Hospice facility / palliative care unit
   12 Acute care hospital
   13 Correctional facility
   14 Other
   15 Deceased

SECTION T. Assessment Information

SIGNATURE OF PERSON COORDINATING / COMPLETING THE ASSESSMENT

_____

1. Signature (sign on above line)

2. Date assessment signed as complete
   2 0 _ _ — _ _ — _ _
   Year   Month   Day